GOING DOWN

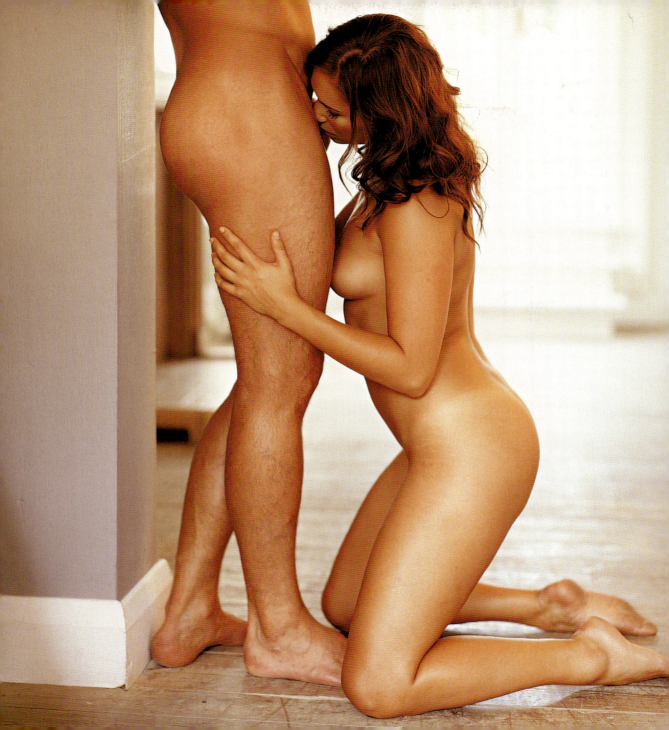

amorata press

GOING DOWN

an illustrated guide to giving him the best blow job of his life

Nicci Talbot

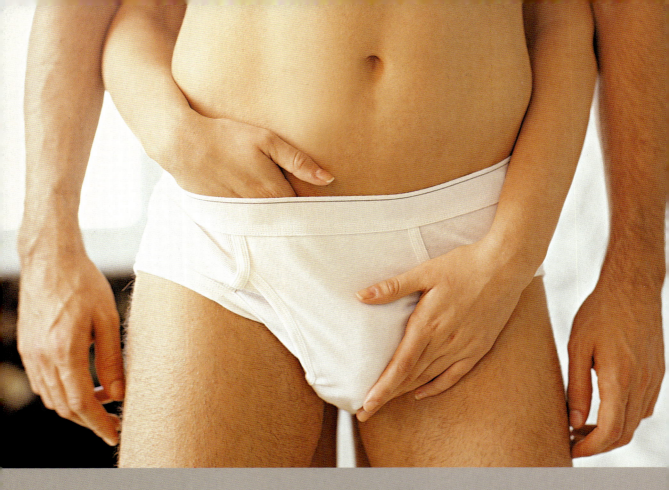

Published in the U.S. by
AMORATA PRESS
P.O. Box 3440
Berkeley, CA 94703
www.amoratapress.com

First published in the U.K. in 2007 as *Unzipped* by Hamlyn, an imprint of Octopus Publishing Group Ltd

Copyright © 2008 Octopus Publishing Group Ltd
Text copyright © 2008 Nicci Talbot

All rights reserved. No part of this work may be reproduced or utilized in any form or by any means, electronic or mechanical, including photocopying, recording or by any information storage and retrieval system, without the prior written permission of the publisher.

Nicci Talbot asserts the moral right to be identified as the author of this work

ISBN-13: 978-1-56975-629-4

Library of Congress Control Number 2007938751

Printed and bound in Hong Kong

10 9 8 7 6 5 4 3

Distributed by Publishers Group West

contents

introduction 6

know his body 18

lip-smackingly good 44

getting in the mood 64

a perfect blow job every time 80

sex play 110

index 124
acknowledgements 128

introduction

Welcome to this book about fellatio. It will inspire and inform you on how to give him the best blow job he's ever had. But believe it or not, there is bad fellatio as well as good, and this book will show you the difference.

It's a myth that most men are so grateful to have a hot mouth wrapped around their privates that they don't care what you do with it. Giving good head is an art – a creative act that requires thought, skill, technique and a little planning. No doubt your partner has had many good blow jobs in his time but by following this guide to develop your skill and technique, you'll make sure that yours are the ones he's begging for.

why do men love it so much?

For many men oral sex is their favourite sexual indulgence. It's an intimate, highly sexy act that feels animalistic. Your lips and tongue provide tonnes of stimulation, sensation and different textures. Plus, your mouth is hot and wet, much like your vagina feels when he's inside you, except your tongue is agile and so can hit just the right spots to thrill him to orgasm.

Spice it up by adjusting the pressure and sensation on a whim or use props like food, drink or sex toys. Most important, though, is the psychological aspect of power exchange – by taking his most vulnerable bits into your mouth, you are accepting all of him, especially if you swallow his come. It's a truly personal, intimate exchange that can tightly bond a couple.

what men say

So, how do you know what men want from a blow job? Well, apart from talking to your partner about it – and that's the best place to start – read on to discover what's hot and what's not on the fellatio front. We polled a few men for their opinion and here's what they said…

having fun

Good fellatio is all about attitude, being in the moment and enjoying yourself. All the tips and techniques in the world can't make up for that. Ask yourself how you feel about oral sex. Does it trigger things for you that you need to work on? What have been your experiences of it so far and have they been enjoyable? Oral sex is far more intimate than intercourse and, as you will soon see, requires a little forethought and practice to do it well. So, if you're feeling exhausted or are simply not in the mood and it's a half-hearted effort then just don't bother. Your partner will be able to tell and it will also put a dampener on it for you both – do something else instead.

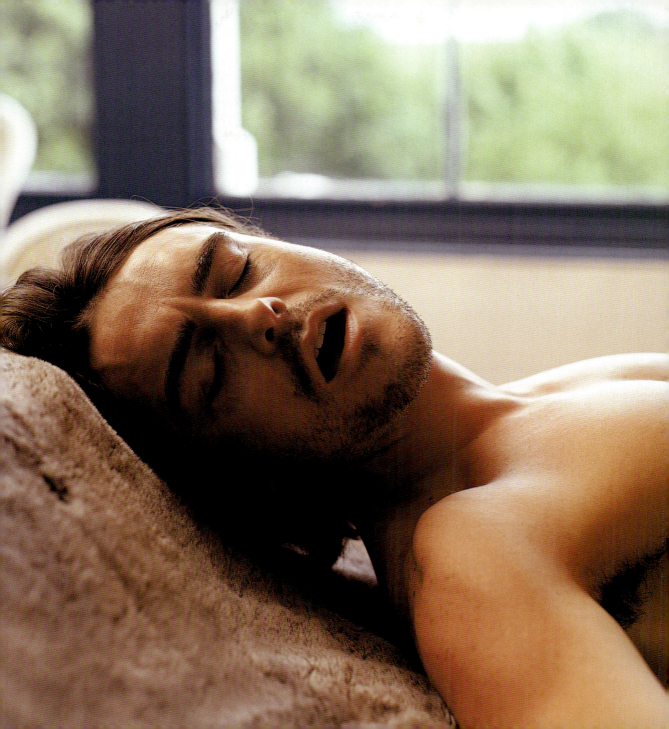

so, what's a spectacular blow job?

'When she keeps me on my toes and I don't know what's coming next.' ... 'A hot, wet mouth and sliding hands.' ... 'Mixing things up – changing tack – slowing down, speeding up – varying her technique.' ... 'It's when she looks at me with sexy eyes like she's hungry for all of me and she just can't get enough.' ... 'It's about attitude, sexiness, fun, playfulness, confidence – the lights are definitely on!' ... 'When she uses her hands and mouth – her whole body – to turn me on and moans her way through it, it's about anticipation – exploring all of my body before she gets to my cock.' ... 'Teasing me until my legs are quivering and I'm begging her to let me come. It's about *her* being in control of my orgasm – and getting herself off on it too.'

and what kind doesn't pass muster?

'Blow jobs that last 20 seconds.' ... 'Being bitten.' ... 'When she'd rather be anywhere else.' ... 'When she's watching the clock or a million miles away – or worse still, scrabbling around for her phone in the middle of it.' ... 'When she stops what she's doing just as I'm about to come.' ... 'When it's the same every time and I know exactly what she's going to do next.'

variety is the spice of life

Don't pressure yourself into becoming Linda 'Deep Throat' Lovelace overnight, give yourself time to try out new tips and discover how your man responds to this new titillation. One of the best approaches is to make just a few small changes to spice up your oral sex life. So, surprise him with a morning session under the covers instead of leaving it until last thing at night for a quick, and no doubt lack-lustre, fumble. It could be as simple as introducing sex toys, erotic food feasts or giving each other a warm-up massage session. If you find that you always use the same strokes because you know what works for him, then mix it up and learn one or two new tricks to keep him guessing and the experience fresh – more on that later (see page 84).

mutual pleasure

A blow job isn't just about your partner's ecstasy and getting him off – it's about your gratification too. If you think of it as something you do for him, then challenge that assumption so that you see yourself as the one in control, deriving pleasure for yourself. It's foreplay, after all, and that involves the two of you.

Why not choose a position to fellate your partner in which you can stimulate yourself (for example, straddling a leg) or demand that he fondles your breasts while you're doing it as a prelude to intercourse? It's the most fabulous power trip to know that you are giving a man the most intense pleasure – and an amazing aphrodisiac. You are in charge of when and how he climaxes: you can make him come quickly – or draw it out and tease him until he begs for mercy.

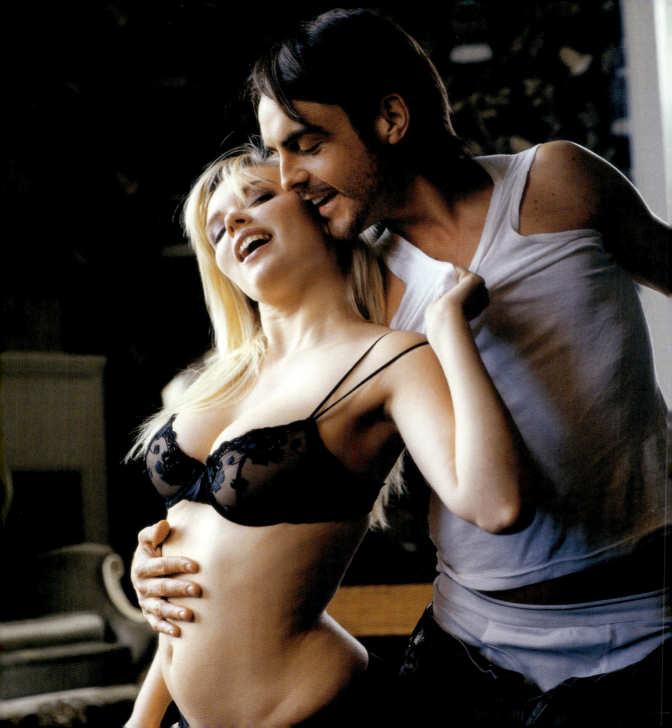

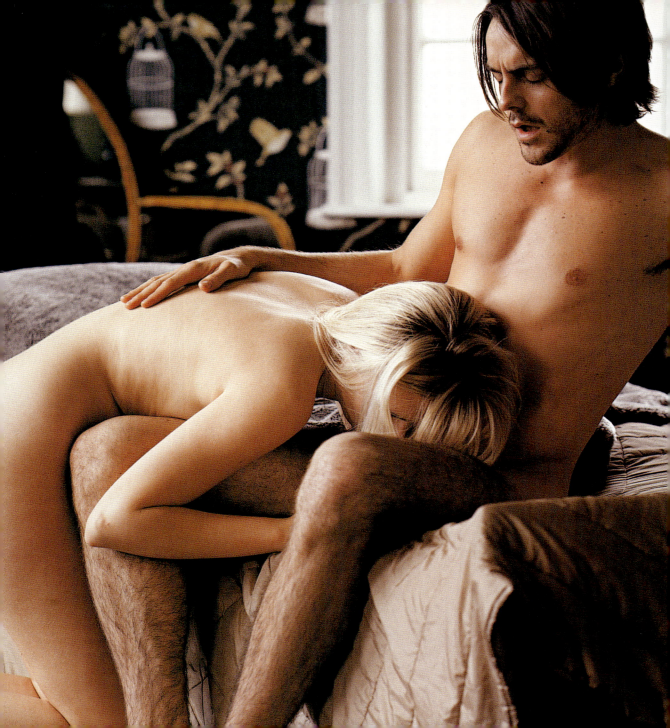

a brief history

Fellatio is the act of licking, sucking, giving a man pleasure or making love with your mouth on his genitals. Slang words for it include 'giving head', 'going down', 'sucking dick' and 'blow job'. The word 'fellatio' itself comes from the Latin word *fellare*, which means 'to suck.'

It's thought that the term 'blow job' came from a prostitute's call to men on the street in the 1930s – 'I'll blow you off' meaning 'I'll help you to blow off steam'. The term is misleading as actually it has nothing to do with blowing a man – although he's sure to appreciate a gentle blow on the tip of the glans after a good licking…

ancient origins

Some say that its origins stem from ancient Egypt and the myth of Osiris and Iris (she breathed life back into his artificial penis). While others put forward the idea that it was introduced as a sexual act by the women of Lesbos (Sapphists), Greece, who used semen to whiten their lips.

It's certainly had its fair share of bad press over the years – the *Kama Sutra*, for example, has an entire chapter on it, describing it in great detail and in part as degrading and unclean, practised by unchaste women and not to be engaged in by men of good standing.

cultural differences

Oral sex is taboo in certain cultures and it is still illegal in around 13 states of the US. Yet, the Taoists in ancient China had no taboos around sexuality and saw it, in fact, as a life-enhancing act. Even a generation ago oral sex wasn't commonly practised. It's only over the past 20 years or so that it has become acceptable and sexual attitudes have mellowed somewhat.

According to a recent study, around 80 per cent of men and women have tried oral sex, although it's more commonly practised by women. For most of us it's a normal part of a healthy and fulfilling sex life and we don't think twice about it. It's a highly intimate, sensual and exciting act that signifies that you accept every bit of your partner and enjoy giving him pleasure.

myths and worries

A few common problems or worries can affect the enjoyment of fellatio. Because it's such an intimate act, communication is key. Talk to your partner and find out what he likes and doesn't like, then say how comfortable you are with fulfilling his desires. Do any of the comments below resonate with you?

he says...
- I'm worried she might bite me.
- I can't relax enough to let go and orgasm.
- I won't let her give me oral sex.
- It's really boring.
- I don't feel able to express myself vocally during oral sex and my partner doesn't know if she's any good at it.

she says...
- His cock is too big for my mouth.
- It's really boring.
- I hate the taste of semen in my mouth.
- I tend to gag or choke.
- I'm afraid he might wee in my mouth.
- I find it degrading and hate the idea of it.
- My jaw locks and I can't open and close my mouth properly.
- My partner is very quiet during oral sex and I have no idea if he likes it or if I'm any good at it.
- Someone once said that I was no good at it and it's knocked my confidence – I don't feel able to initiate it.
- I can make my boyfriend come but I always do the same thing now I know what works for him! It's getting boring.
- He doesn't reciprocate so why should I go to the effort to please him if he won't return the favour?
- He sometimes loses his erection when I'm doing it and I wonder if it's my technique.
- I don't like the taste and smell of his genitals.
- I'm worried about catching an STI.
- I can't make him come no matter what I do.
- I hate the feeling of pubes in my mouth.

These are all perfectly normal and common responses to fellatio but if you're worried about something in particular or don't feel able to discuss it with your partner, then consider talking to a counsellor or sex therapist – they can give you a different perspective on things and help you to work things through.

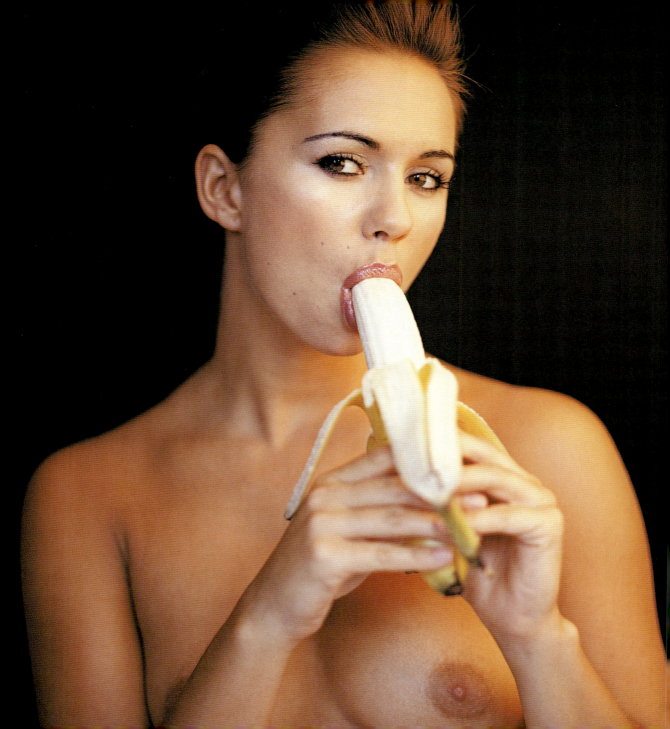

safe sex

Both giving and receiving oral sex can be risky activities, for example if a partner has a sexually transmitted infection (STI) or if you don't know each other's sexual history. Oral sex is a much lower risk activity than intercourse but there is still the risk of transmission. So, if in doubt use protection and practise safe oral sex.

common STIs

Sexually transmitted infections can be passed on via the mouth or in sexual fluids; some STIs can be transmitted in the rare case of blood being present during oral sex (hepatitis B) or via faeces (hepatitis A).

The most common STIs are:

- chlamydia
- gonorrhoea
- hepatitis A (via rimming or licking the anal area)
- hepatitis B
- hepatitis C (only via blood transmission)
- herpes type 1 (which leads to cold sores)
- herpes type 2 (which leads to genital herpes)
- HIV
- human papilloma virus (HPV)
- syphilis

The risk of HIV infection is greater for the person performing the oral sex than the receiver. There's a small risk of HIV – it can occur if sexual fluid or blood gets into a cut, sore or ulcer in the mouth or throat. Some experts advise not brushing your teeth before oral sex as it can lead to small cuts in the mouth.

get it on

Stay safe and use condoms and dental dams (rectangular sheets of latex) for oral play and oral–anal play. Barriers such as these are widely used in the States and their popularity is increasing round the world. In the UK, prostitutes now use condoms as standard for fellatio (incidentally, it's their most popular request).

to swallow or not

You're more at risk if your partner comes in your mouth so unless you're using condoms don't let him ejaculate directly into your mouth, especially if he is a new partner or you are unsure of his sexual history. Men often grumble that condoms ruin their sensation and the spontaneity of sex but that doesn't have to be the case. You simply need to experiment with different types, use lubricants and learn how to eroticize putting a condom on to make it an exciting part of your foreplay (see pages 63, 114–117).

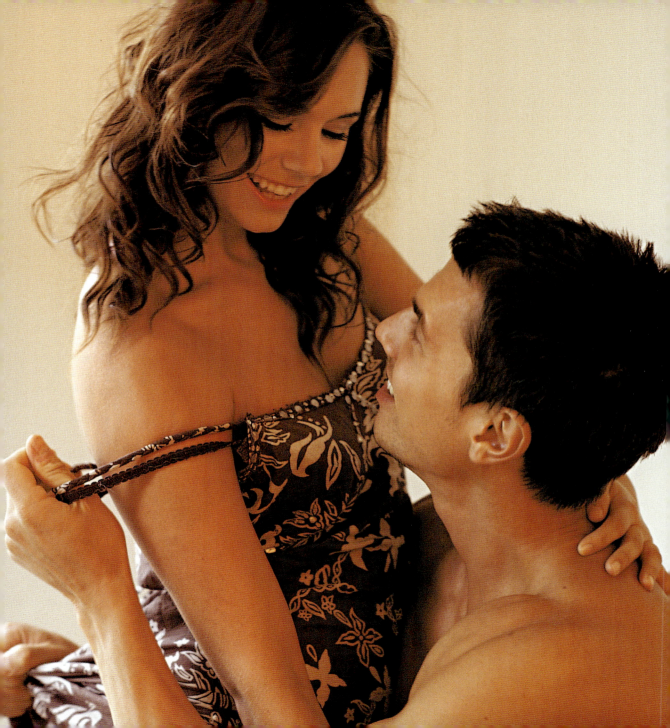

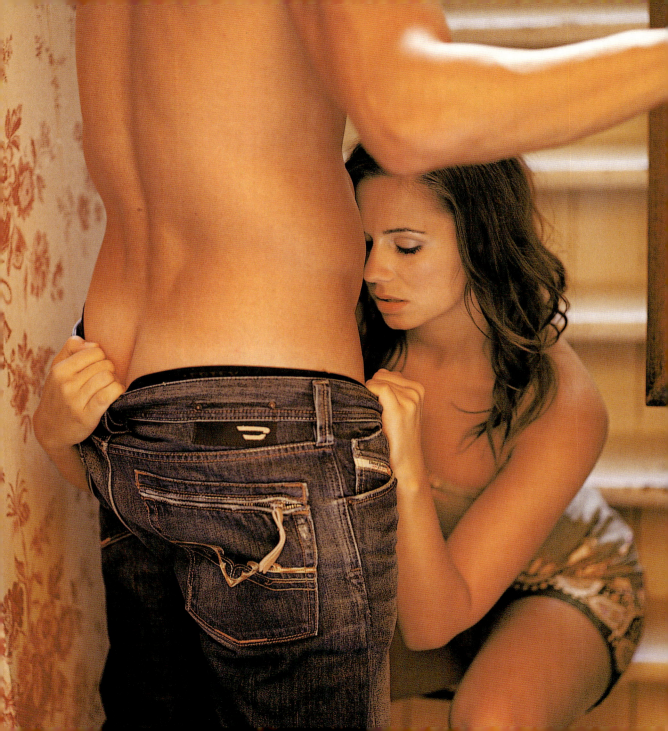

how to use the book

This book is divided into five parts so that you can dip in and out according to what you'd like to know. Read on to discover whether you should skip straight to one particular section or leaf through others on the way.

know his body
Part 1 is all about his body and how the penis works – a brief lesson in anatomy if you don't already know what you're working with. Knowing how his arousal cycle works, too, will give you more confidence so that oral sex becomes more fulfilling for you both.

lip-smackingly good
Part 2 is all about you – your facial anatomy, how the jaw, tongue and mouth function, with a few fun exercises thrown in to get your mouth into training and make performing fellatio a more comfortable experience for you.

getting in the mood
Part 3 explores foreplay and why it's so important. Of course, oral sex is part of foreplay and there are many other things you can do to make sex more exhilarating and indulgent, such as erotic massage, feasting off each other's bodies and cuddling – closeness is key.

a perfect blow job every time
Explore the different tried-and-tested positions and techniques and try out some of the new tricks or keep some up your sleeve and surprise him. If time is short, there are a few tips on quickies, as well as how to tease and titillate your man and build-up to an explosive orgasm. And happy endings – how to finish a blow job properly and what to do if you don't want to swallow.

sex play
The final part of the book takes a look at how sex toys and body modification can add a little extra something to your oral adventures.

the journey is about to begin
Every man has his quirks and no two cocks are the same, so you may well need to adapt your techniques to suit your partner – but that's what makes blow jobs exciting, you constantly experiment. The thrill is in the journey and orgasm shouldn't be seen as the end – and only – goal.

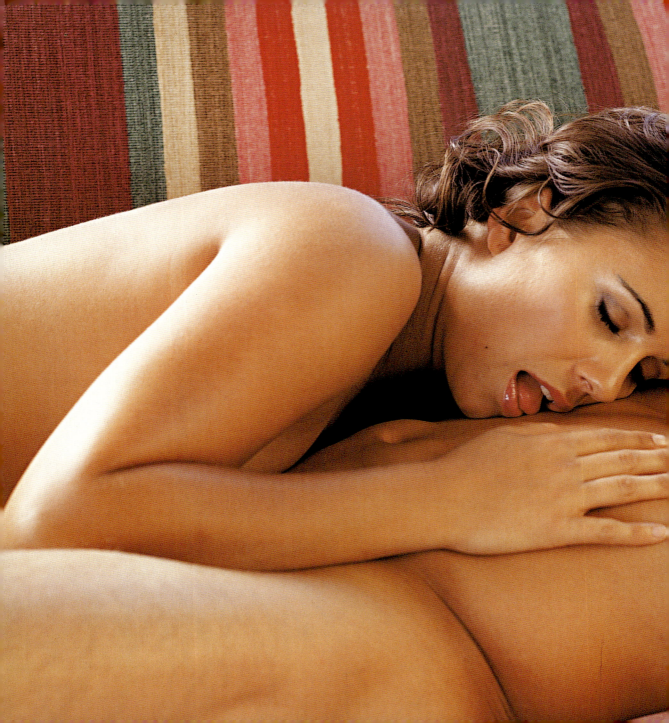

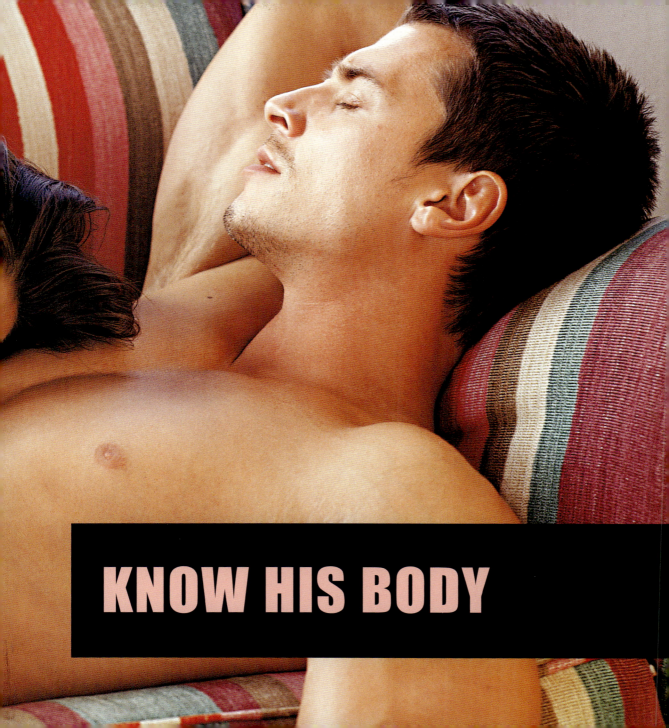

know his body

In this section we're going to look at how his body works – his penis specifically. But although his penis takes centre stage, you'd be foolish to concentrate on it exclusively and ignore other hot spots. Paying a little attention to his erogenous zones (he may not even know where they are!) will intensify the experience for you both – and make his orgasm even stronger. Knowing a bit about his anatomy along with his sexual response cycle is the first step in improving your technique. You'll know what bits to press and why, so to speak.

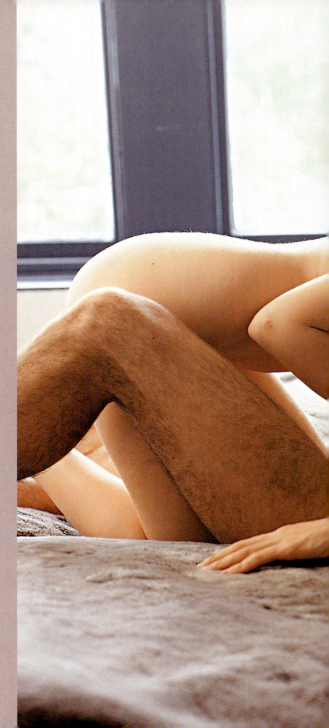

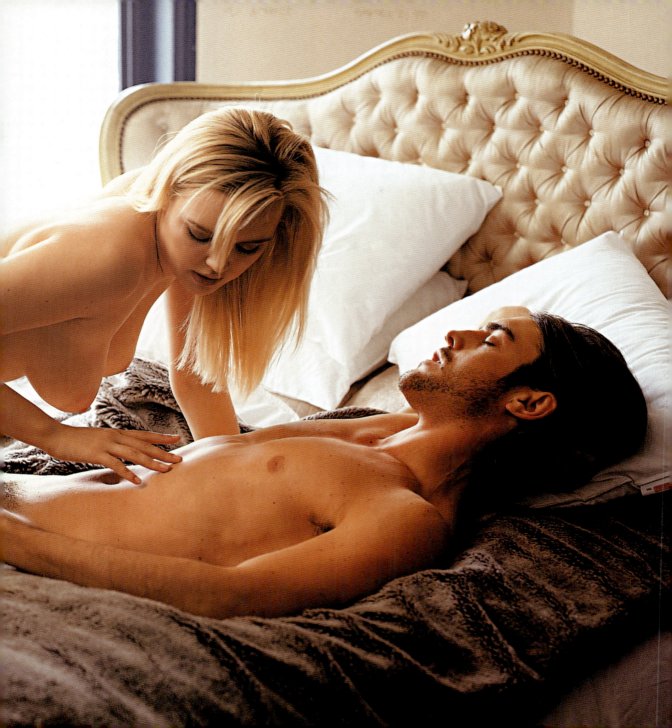

take a long, hard look

If you want to improve your technique then get to know his genitals intimately, so that you can push the right buttons to rock his world.

first things first
Get your partner to undress – or strip him off and get him to lie down on the bed. Make sure the room is warm and that he is relaxed and comfortable. Now, take a look at his penis – it might sound a bit strange, but how many times have you examined it closely?

take hold
Warm up your hands and hold his cock between them. Notice the texture, the hair, the softness and firmness, and how it swells. Move your fingers along the underside of his penis, next to his belly, and explore this area for hot spots. Notice the scrotum and his testicles, and how snug they are to his body – moving closer and higher as he gets harder. Behind his scrotum is another sensitive area – known as the million-dollar point (see page 30).

the angle of dangle
Does his penis bend to one side when erect? If so, adapt positions for oral sex to suit. Cup his testicles in your hands. They can be extremely sensitive, so go slowly to discover how he likes them handled. Massage them if you want to slow him down.

pushing the button
The fleshy mound of skin that covers his pubic bone is full of sensitive spots. Gently massage it with the heel of your hand to stimulate blood flow. His perineum – the smooth bit between his penis and his anus – is where his penis root is; you can feel it harden as his erection grows. Gently explore his anal area, the lightest touch here reaps massive ecstatic rewards.

> **try this!**
> *Watch his body language and breathing. What makes him breathe heavier? Does he have goosebumps when you touch certain areas? (More on reading his body in Part 4, pages 80–109.)*

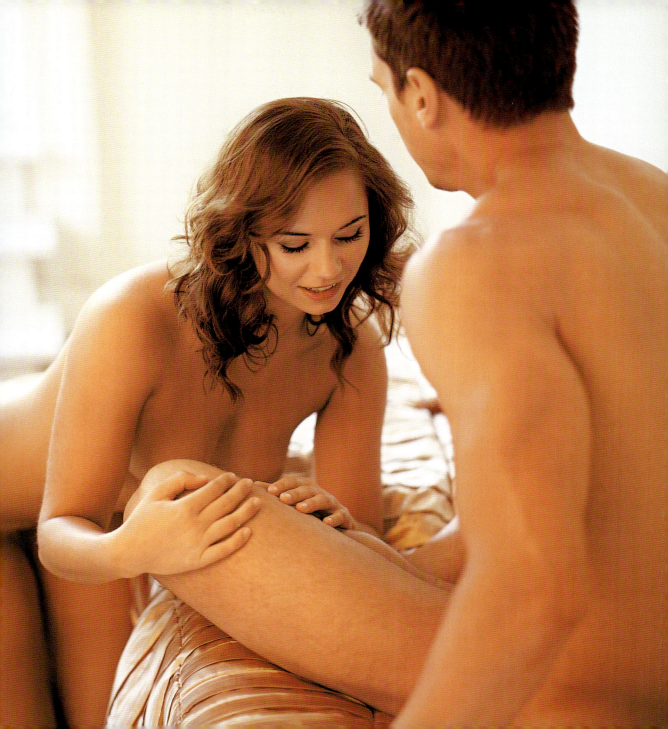

a user's guide

His penis is a marvellous piece of machinery. No two are the same shape nor do they like to be handled in the same way. That's what makes oral sex such an adventure. Now you're a bit more familiar with your partner's penis, unearth all the different parts and learn how to make the most of them.

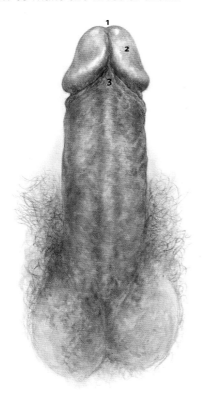

the penis
His cock is packed with blood vessels and erectile tissue. Over the glans (the head of the penis), the skin forms a fold – the foreskin – and his urethra lies deep within. Penises come in all shapes and sizes, colours and textures. The average size of an erect penis is 13–16 cm (5–7 in) long with a girth of about 10 cm (4 in). And since your mouth cavity is around 9 cm (3½ in) deep you can see why deepthroating is pretty tricky!

1 the meatus
This tiny opening in the top of the glans lets out urine and semen. Not at the same time, though – if he's ejaculating the entrance to the bladder is closed off so that the two substances never mix.

2 the glans
The head of his penis is the most sensitive part. Find out how he likes to be handled – the level of pressure will be determined by his sensitivity. Immediately after orgasm the glans is usually too sensitive to touch and many men prefer no further stimulation.

3 the frenulum
This V-shaped notch at the back of the glans feels slightly ridged in texture. This and the coronal ridge (where the seam of the glans meets the shaft) are the hot spots. For an ultra-fast orgasm, lick or flutter your tongue around this part.

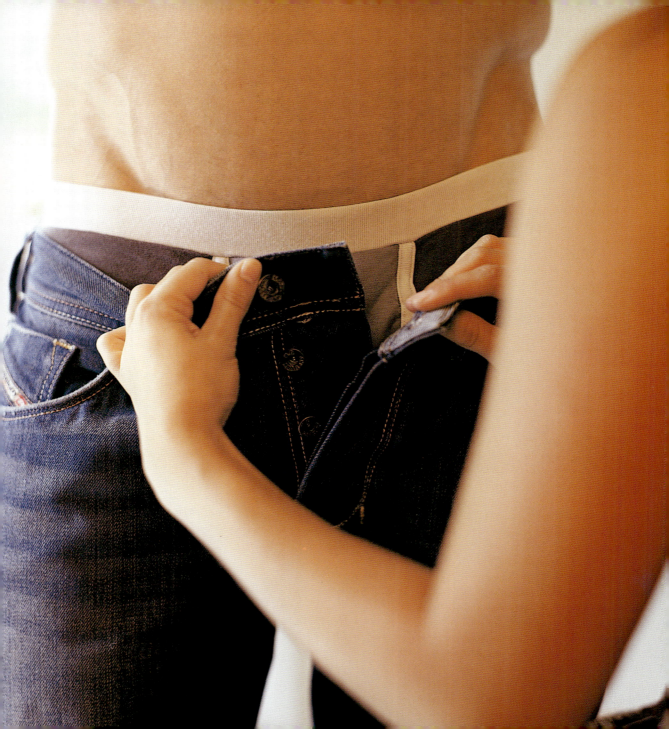

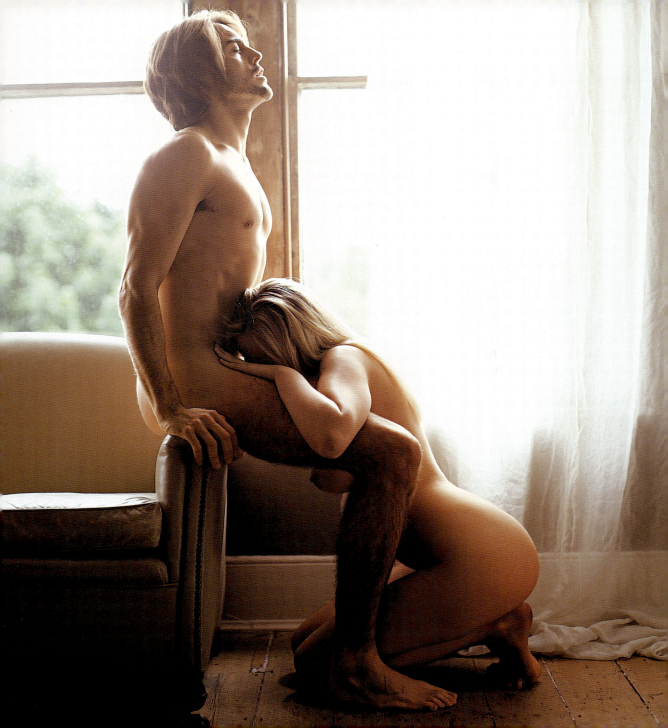

how to handle his penis

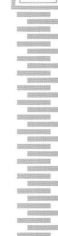

Men sometimes say that women are too gentle when they handle their penis. Don't be tempted to go to the other extreme, though, and get too rough (unless he likes it!). Most guys like a fair amount of pressure (older men need more pressure than younger ones) but you'll need to find the right level for your partner.

start on the shaft

Make him feel good by increasing the pressure and speed on his shaft. The underbelly of the shaft is a hot spot, so a long lick here, from bottom to top, will emphasize his length and feel sensational. Now, take the shaft between your hands and glide them along his skin. Or for a sexy alternative, take his cock in your mouth when flaccid and feel it swell, as he gets more excited.

faster and harder

Once he's erect you can move faster, and harder, too, if he likes it, and slip into a rhythm. Rhythm is vital in bringing him to orgasm. It's okay to tease, and stop and start at the beginning but once he's close to climax keep a continual rhythm. When he comes, he experiences rhythmic muscle contractions so replicating that pulsing movement with your hands or your mouth will intensify his orgasm no end.

what rocks his world?

If you're not sure what he likes then ask him outright. You could get him to masturbate for you – and then you can join in. It's incredibly sexy for both of you to be intimately sharing this knowledge. Spend time on the glans – his route to nirvana. As well as being hands-on, lick or suck it gently, manipulate the foreskin with your tongue, roll it around in your cheeks and then hold it in your mouth for a while.

> ### try this!
> *If your man loses his erection during oral sex, just shift the focus or change the pressure. Move away from his penis and pay attention to the rest of his body, but especially his scrotum and testicles. Create anticipation and then switch back to his penis.*

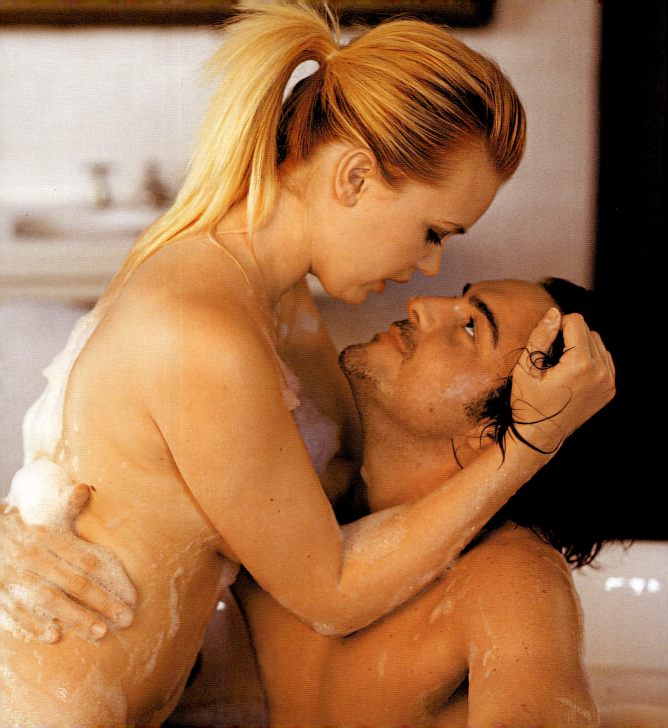

common concerns

If you have a worry that is getting in the way of giving your partner oral pleasure then take comfort that you are not alone. Common anxieties include not liking the smell of his genitals, watching as his erection wilts before your eyes and wondering if all men get hard at the same speed. Read on to quell your anxieties and find out what to try instead.

smells down there

Everyone has their own personal smell (and taste). Even when someone washes every day, dirt and sweat can build up and produce a 'cheesy' odour called smegma if he's uncut. His genitals are his core and how they taste and smell varies according to his health, lifestyle, diet and stress levels. If you're not keen on fellating your man because of the smell down there be honest with him and talk about it. Suggest you shower together as a prelude to oral sex. Encourage him to wash behind his foreskin – or do it for him.

waxing and waning erection

It's normal for his penis to rise and fall during stimulation, and that doesn't mean that he's not in seventh heaven. But perhaps the position you're choosing to fellate him in is contributing to the 'problem'. Gravity can sometimes affect his erection so if he's on his back get him to turn over onto his knees; or ask him to stand or lean against something. Try the positions on pages 93–105.

are all erections equal?

Do all men get hard at the same speed? When your man is excited his penis fills with blood, causing an erection. The blood is then trapped there for a while to prevent him losing his hardness. Younger men may have more frequent, quicker or harder erections than older men. According to the Taoists, there are four stages of erection: firmless/lengthening; swelling; hardness; and heat (when he's about to ejaculate). Doctors in the West have acknowledged these stages but they have more formal ways to describe the physiological changes (see His sexual response, page 39).

hot spots down below

Now you're on intimate terms with your partner's penis, you can start to pay some attention to the many other hot spots down below. And get some great tips on the way.

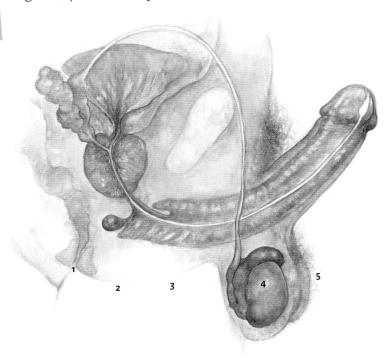

1 the anus
The anus is packed with nerve endings. You'll be able to stimulate his prostate gland (his G-spot equivalent) via this area (see page 33).

2 the million-dollar point
This hot spot, according to the Taoists, is on the perineal area close to the anus. In contrast to the perineum, though, pressing on this point promotes blood flow into the penis and can help slow down ejaculation.

3 the perineum
This is the smooth, flat bit of skin between his testicles and his anus. It's a super-hot spot and a little sustained pressure here when he's having an orgasm will intensify things.

4 the testicles
Each testicle produces sperm and testosterone. As he's about to ejaculate, the scrotum contracts and hugs the testicles close to his body. So, a delaying tactic is to pull them away from his body before he comes.

5 the scrotum
This sac hangs beneath his penis and houses his testicles. Some men like it when you gently tug it during fellatio.

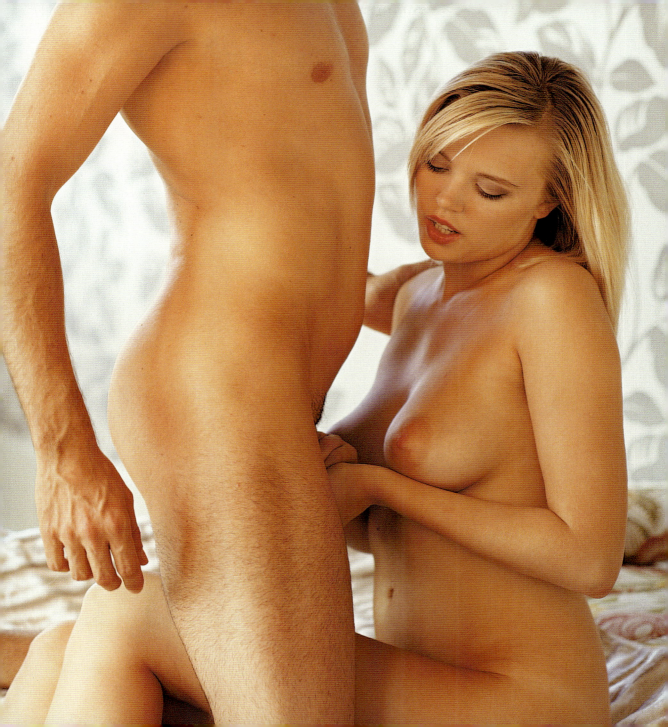

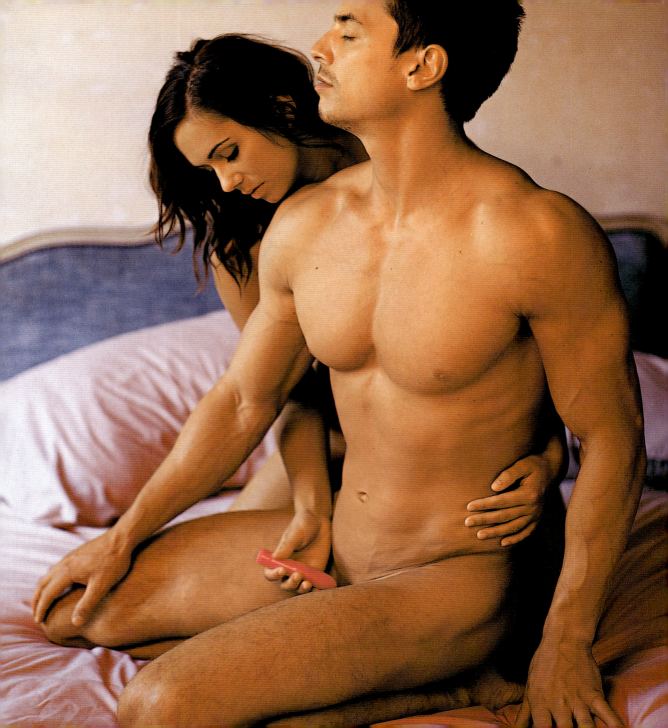

hidden from view

Your man's reproductive equipment is truly impressive. As well as making millions of sperm every day, along with all that they need to survive the journey into the vagina and beyond, his genitals can respond in an instant to stimulation to be ready for action. If you're interested in internally massaging your partner then read on.

the prostate gland

This gland secretes substances into semen as the fluid passes through on its way from the seminal vesicles to the urethra. It's located under the bladder and in front of the rectum. You can think of it as his G-spot.

Stimulating his prostate can give him a huge amount of pleasure and an intense orgasm. What's more, 'milking' his prostate via internal massage keeps his prostate healthy! As with women, it seems that men have more than one orgasm – one from the prostate and the other from his penis. Men report that a prostate orgasm feels deeper, lasts longer, is more intense than a regular orgasm and the waves ripple through their entire body, not just their genitals.

Get him to lie back with his knees up while you kneel in front of him. Once he's aroused, you can stimulate his prostate by gently inserting a lubricated finger or a prostate stimulator toy into his anus. Curve your finger towards yourself (as if making the 'come hither' motion) once it's inside his anus until you can feel a ridged area. The more aroused he is the bigger it becomes, which is why it's a good idea to wait until he's turned on before attempting it. It's best to press on it rather than sliding your finger in and out as direct pressure feels exquisite.

pubococcygeus (pc) muscle

His PC muscle, running between his pubic bone and his coccyx, has a vital sexual function. If he whips this muscle into shape his orgasms will be more intense and, what's more, he'll recover more quickly. Blood will flow more freely in his pelvis so he will be more responsive to touch. In addition, he will be able to learn how to separate orgasm from ejaculation. The easiest way to identify the muscle is to stop and start your urine flow when you're on the toilet. If both of you practise several times daily you'll soon notice a massive improvement in your sex life.

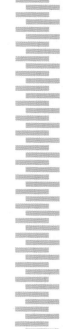

1 the vas deferens
This tube passes from the epididymis up and around the bladder before entering the prostate gland, where it connects to a tube from the seminal vesicle to form the ejaculatory duct. Sperm moves along this tube before he ejaculates.

2 the prostate gland
It secretes substances into semen as the fluid passes through on its way from the seminal vesicles to the urethra. It's located under the bladder and in front of the rectum.

3 the corpa cavernosa
The two cylindrical bodies of erectile tissue lie on either side of the penis. The spongy nature of the tissue allows them to become rigid when the penis fills with blood, causing his erection.

4 the epididymis
His sperm cells mature and sit in this long coiled tube that runs along the back of his testicle until he ejaculates during orgasm.

5 cowper's glands
Along with the prostate, these glands produce his pre-ejaculate – the tiny drops of fluid that appear on his glans just before he ejaculates. Pre-come does contain sperm, which is why the withdrawal method isn't recommended as a contraceptive.

6 the ejaculatory ducts
Semen moves through these when he comes.

7 the seminal vesicles
A pair of sacs behind the bladder that produce the seminal fluid, which is mixed with sperm to make semen.

> ### try this!
> If you're worried about hygiene or want to practise safer oral sex then consider using a dental dam. It's highly unlikely you'll encounter any faeces during internal stimulation, but if you prefer you could learn how to give him an enema to 'clean him out' internally.

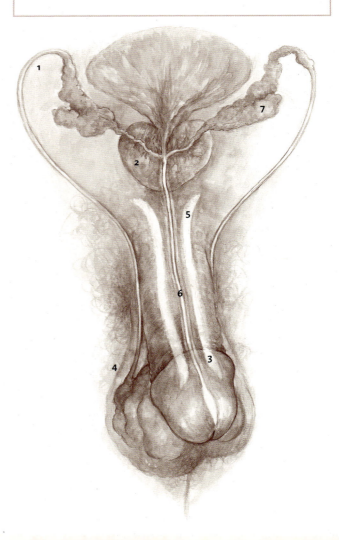

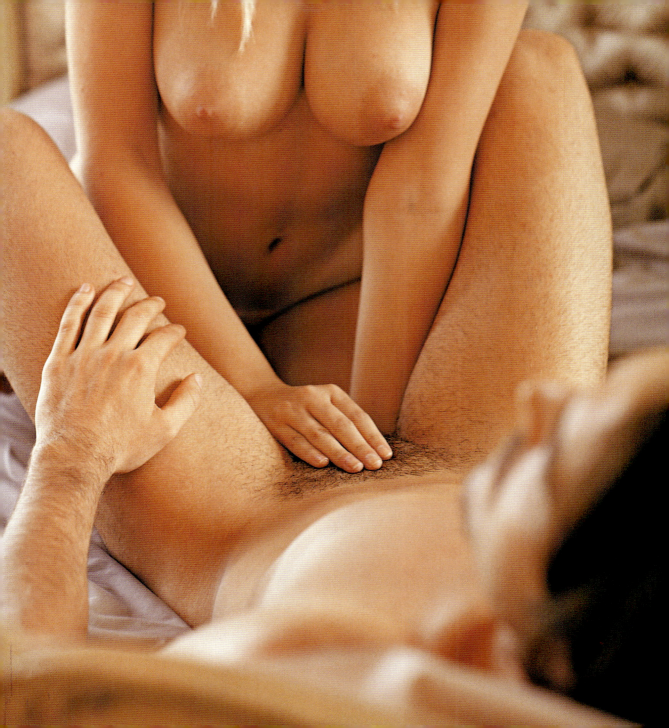

anatomy of ejaculation

It's easy to think of orgasm and ejaculation as the same thing but they are, in fact, two separate stages, although they generally happen around the same time. Orgasm refers to the muscular contraction that occurs at 0.8-second intervals, while the ejaculation is the expulsion of semen from his penis. The average ejaculate measures less than a teaspoon of fluid (1–5 ml) – less than you might think when it's spurted into your mouth!

It's important to know that orgasm and ejaculation are two separate processes because if your partner can learn how to separate the two and orgasm without ejaculating, he can experience multiple orgasms. Ejaculation is depleting – often the reason he feels the need to sleep right after sex.

what's in ejaculate?

Semen is pretty healthy stuff – it contains about 15 kcal per ejaculation. It's mostly water (90 per cent) along with semen from the seminal vesicles and the prostate gland; the latter's contribution is said to give it its characteristic smell. One load of ejaculate contains 40–60 million sperm as well as mood-enhancing hormones. Furthermore, it contains the following ingredients in tiny quantities that help to protect and nurture the sperm on its journey to that elusive egg: aboutonia, ascorbic acid, blood-group antigens, calcium, chloride, cholesterol, choline, citric acid, creatine, deoxyribonucleic acid, fructose, glutathione, hyaluronidase, inositol, lactic acid, magnesium, nitrogen, phosphorus, potassium, purine, pyramidine, pyruvic acid, sodium, sorbitol, spermadine, spermine, urea, uric acid, vitamin B12, and zinc.

it's actually good for you!

You might scoff at the porn shots where a man comes all over a woman's face or chest yet it's arousing for him to see and semen is actually good for your skin – it moisturizes, firms and softens it. Just remember to close your eyes, as it can sting. The taste of semen varies according to how long its been since his last ejaculation and what he's eaten, so you can change it by making a few tweaks to his diet (see page 73).

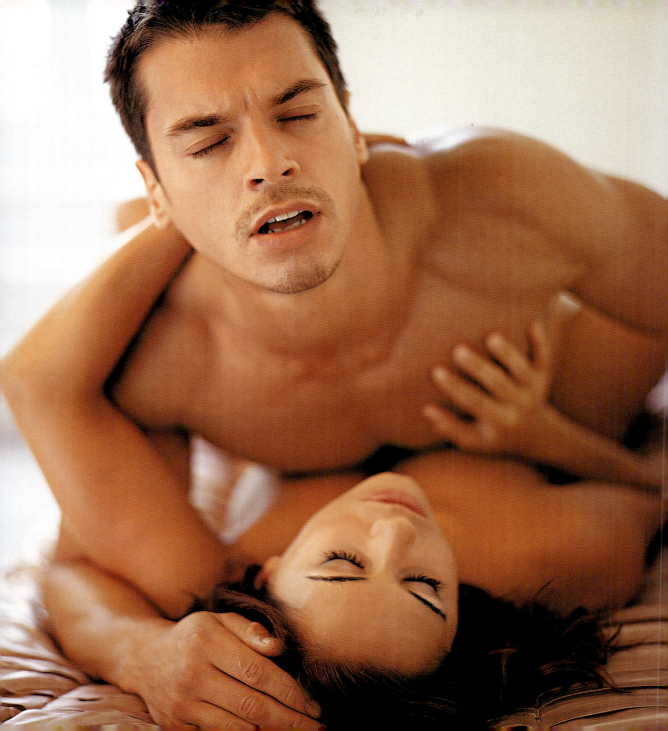

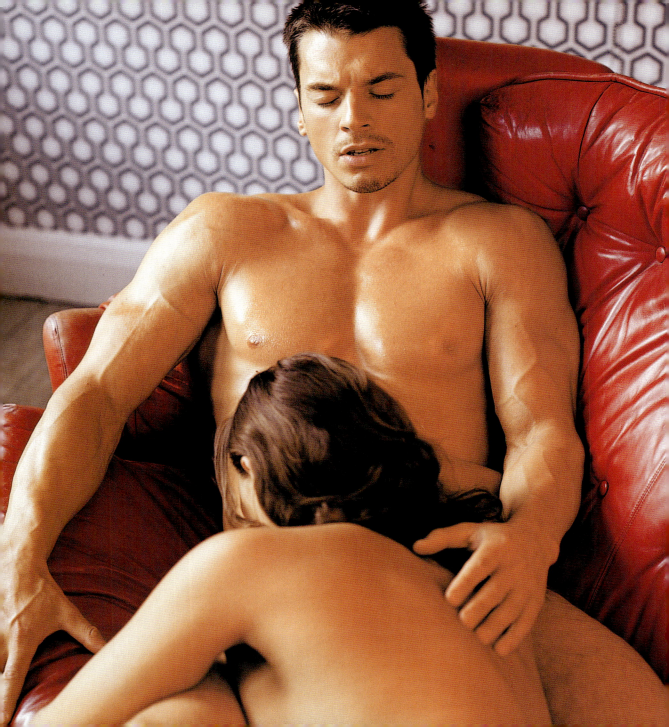

his sexual response

Sexologists Masters and Johnson defined four stages of physiological response during sexual stimulation, outlining roughly what happens to his body from the moment he thinks about sex to his orgasm and immediately afterwards. It's useful to know the sexual response cycle as a guideline to what happens but his responses can vary according to his mood, stress, lifestyle and even how he feels about you as a partner.

excitement

Stimulation can be mental or physical – he has a kinky thought or is being aroused by kissing or touch. As a response, his brain triggers an increase in blood flow to certain areas and his body gears itself up for sex. His heart rate and breathing rate soar and blood pressure rises. His nipples have a mini-erection and his skin will flush and start to sweat – the rosy glow that moves up from the tummy to the chest.

Once his brain registers that he's turned on it sends a message to his penis: blood flows to the tissues, making him erect; although his hardness can come and go. His testicles hug his body and his scrotum thickens.

This excitement process is generally much quicker for a man than a woman – it can happen after 10–30 seconds of stimulation in a man whereas women can take anything up to 45 minutes to feel really turned on.

the plateau

This stage is the period just before orgasm. His heart rate and circulation increase further and his whole body becomes ultra-sensitive to touch. His plateau will be slightly longer than yours, although his excitement phase is much shorter. The muscles at the base of the penis contract, the glans swells and his testicles sit even more snugly next to his body. By this point, his heart rate has doubled – to about 180 beats per minute.

orgasm

His body explodes into orgasm, releasing the build up of tension. Both of you experience contractions in the anus and pelvic areas at around 0.8 seconds apart. His body spasms and his orgasm lasts around 5 seconds – slightly less than yours. During orgasm he produces testosterone, which helps to protect his heart – so sex is really good for you. As we mentioned earlier (see page 36) the processes of orgasm and ejaculation are separate, so he is able to come without experiencing ejaculation if he learns how to control it through exercise and breathing. When he's about to come his cock throbs and his scrotum will be snug to his body. His pelvic muscles contract moving fluid through the urethra to spurt out from the meatus. His come can spurt, on average, 17–25 cm (7–10 in). The ejaculate load depends on his age, health and how long it's been since his last orgasm.

resolution

After orgasm his muscles relax, and his breathing and blood pressure return to normal. He'll be blissfully shattered thanks to the release of the hormone prolactin from the pituitary gland in his brain. Resolution is pretty quick for him. He goes into his refractory period (the time he needs to recover before he can orgasm again) and his penis becomes limp and shrinks to half its erect size. His balls drop, too, and soon he'll be asleep. The length of his refractory period depends on his age and general health: the younger he is the quicker his recovery time and the sooner he can be up and ready for more action.

common problems

Common problems with male sexual response include premature ejaculation, which affects over 40 per cent of men, and erectile dysfunction or impotence, which affects at least one in 10 men. If your partner is worried about any of these problems and it's affecting the quality of your sex life, then he should see his doctor first of all in order to rule out any physical causes such as diabetes, deficient blood flow to the penis or hormonal abnormalities. Drinking too much alcohol and using drugs (legal and illegal) can also affect his sexual response. Psychological causes include stress or worry about work or relationships, mood, thoughts, depression, poor self-esteem and previous sexual experiences. It could be a combination of both factors. Most problems are treatable and your doctor will be able to advise on the best course of action.

> **try this!**
> *Pelvic floor (Kegel) exercises can help manage impotence and premature ejaculation and will massively improve his sexual response and orgasms. These exercises can help strengthen the muscles around the penis and also improve blood circulation, which leads to stronger erections. He can identify the muscles by either stopping himself from breaking wind or stopping the flow of urine. Practise squeezing the muscles 10–15 times, holding for 5 seconds then swap and do them faster, letting the muscles drop immediately. Alternate between the two. Once he knows where the muscles are he can practise these exercises at anytime. If you both get into the habit of doing the exercises several times each day you'll soon notice a massive difference in your sexual response after three months or so.*

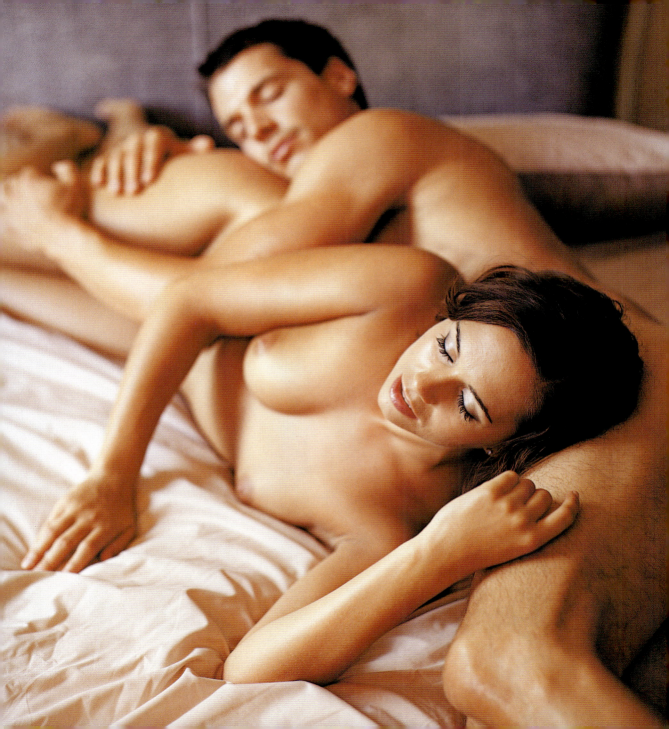

what about the rest?

A truly great blow job doesn't focus just on his penis. To give him a powerful orgasm you need to arouse and excite other body parts first. This is why foreplay is vital. You're waking up his whole body and engaging all of his senses. You might find that he's sensitive in the most unlikely of areas – the armpit, for example!

the skin
Our skin is our largest erogenous zone. Explore his body by kissing, sucking, stroking and nibbling. Vary the pressure from gentle to rough to keep him on his toes, and mix it up by warming his skin with massage oil or cooling it down with ice.

the nipples
Yes, men have them too and they can be highly sensitive if tweaked or sucked during oral sex to help him come to climax. Why not reach up and circle them with your fingertips and tug them gently before you get to his penis or while you're fellating him. If it does nothing for him the first few times, then persist as the nipple tissue swells as he gets excited and becomes more sensitive.

the stomach
Run your hand or mouth down his linea alba – the 'white line' that runs between the right and the left muscles. Start soft and slow, and build up to a more firm massage.

the inner thighs and buttocks
As an area that's often ignored, touching him here will feel extra sexy to him. Start with slow massage strokes and then gently nibble up his thighs. Try a firmer massage on his bum cheeks then gently spread them and massage his inner cheeks from top to bottom.

fingers and toes
Try sucking, licking and biting his fingertips and toes gently. Ask him to suck your fingers the way he'd like you to suck his penis. He'll either love foot massage or hate it – some men are too sensitive.

head and scalp
Most men love having their scalp rubbed and your fingers run through his hair. Give him a scalp massage in the bath when you're washing his hair and use an essential oil like rosemary to get his circulation flowing.

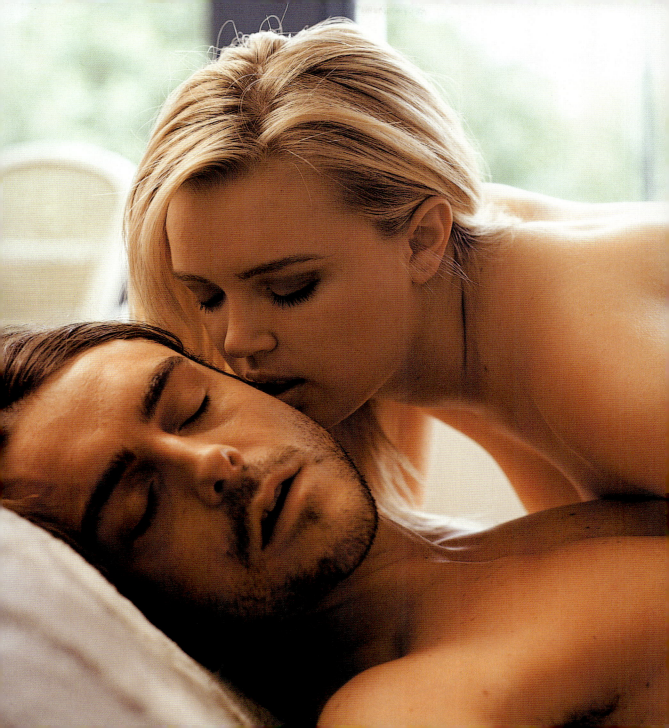

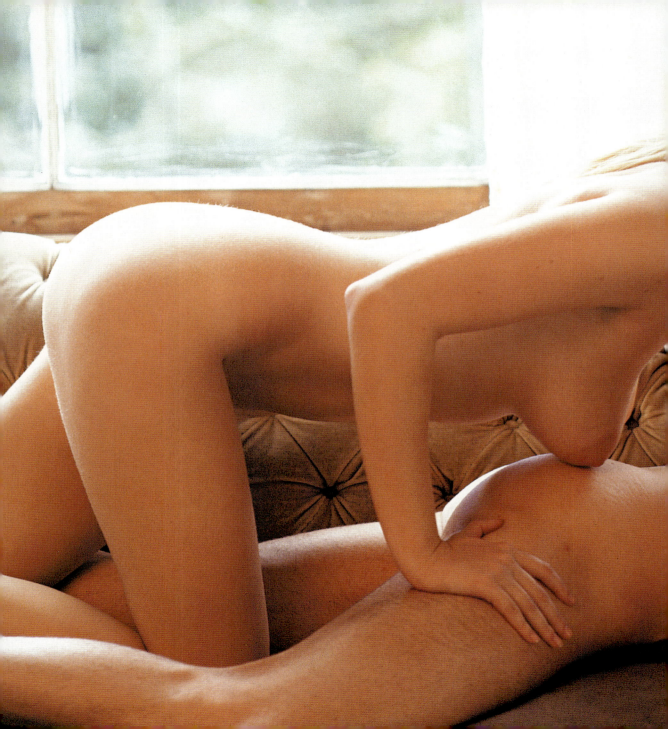

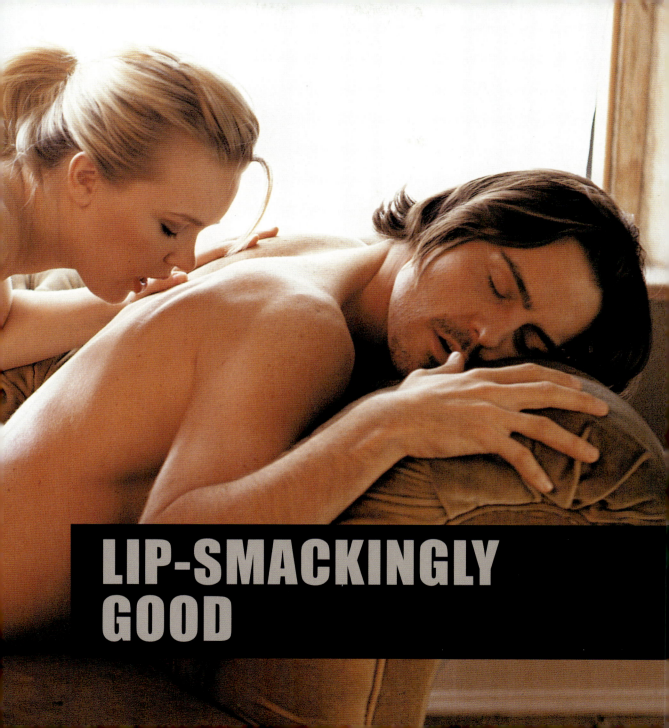

lip-smackingly good

46

You may well not have given much thought to how your mouth, lips, tongue and jaw work – but for great oral technique, a little effort here is a must. So, this section looks at your facial anatomy; once you understand how it all works, you can improve its function. Plus, there are some exercises to strengthen your tongue and relax your jaw and throat muscles. And we're throwing in a few extra pointers on breathing techniques – an essential part of giving good head is being able to breathe easily through your nose – and on how to go about practising these beforehand.

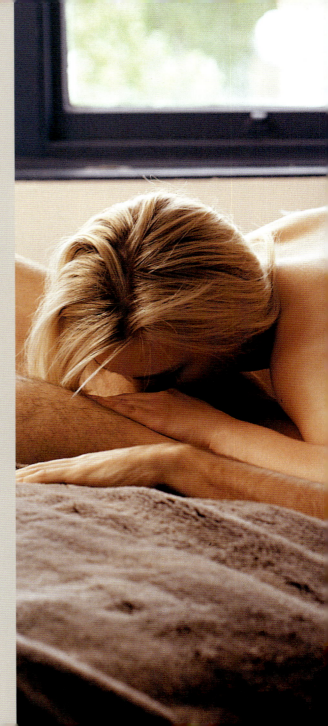

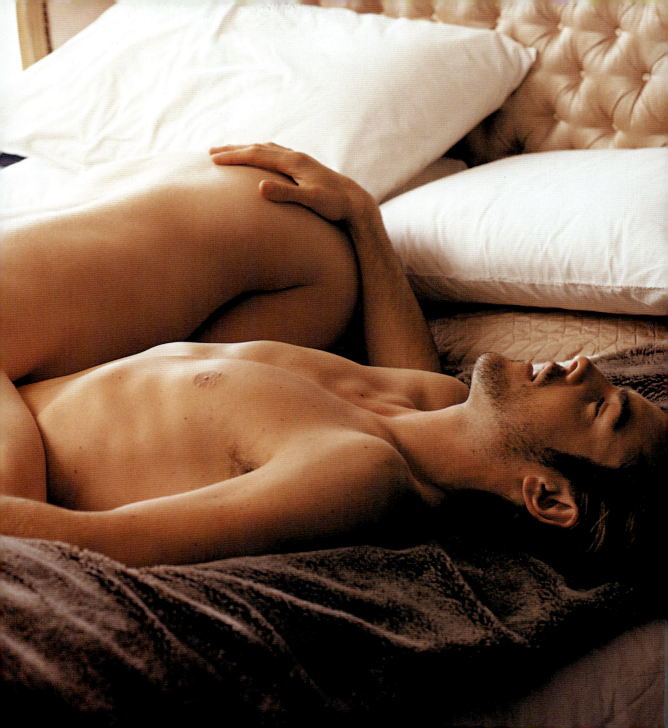

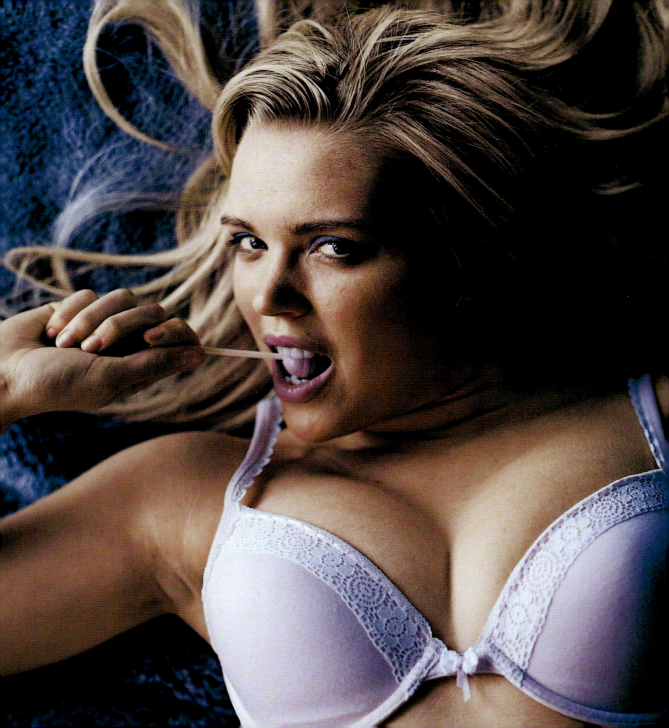

you and your hot mouth

Your face has 14 bones, which enable you to do such varied things as taste, smell, see and hear. Two maxillae bones make up your upper jaw and the mandible bone comprises the lower jaw. The mandible works with the temporal bone (of your skull) to enable your mouth to open and close. Now, what's going on inside?

what the tongue can do

Oral sex is a perfectly natural, instinctive act in which you're exploring surfaces with your tongue. Because it contains many different muscles, you can exercise them to strengthen your tongue and improve your oral technique. Your tongue allows you to taste and to speak, but its highly agile and versatile nature enables you to deliver wonderful sensations during oral sex.

The upper surface of the tongue is covered in tiny bumps called papillae, which give it a rougher texture compared with the smoother surface on the underside.

Your tongue is incredibly sensitive – in fact, it's far more sensitive than your fingers, so it makes perfect sense that you use it to give and to receive oral pleasure. Use your tongue to sense the nuances of his body that you might not be able to pick up through your hands.

taste sensations

The papillae contain our taste buds, which respond to only one type of flavour – salty, bitter, sweet or sour. You taste these flavours on different parts of your tongue: sweet on the tip; salty on the sides near the front; sour on the sides; and bitter at the back, towards the throat. The more taste buds you have, the more intensely you perceive tastes, especially bitter ones. If you like to swallow but don't always like the taste, it's worth using foods during fellatio to counter any bitterness.

> ### try this!
> *Give up smoking as it reduces your ability to taste properly. What's more it leads to a 'flabby' tongue that isn't as capable of quick and agile movements. So, quit today – not only will it make a difference to your general health, but your sex life will benefit too.*

a tongue workout

Your tongue is amazingly agile. This muscular organ responds well to a workout, so practising a few simple exercises can help both to sensitize and to strengthen your tongue. Try some of the specific techniques (see pages 90 and 100) with your new, improved 'tongue power' – your man will be crying out for more.

the rough and the smooth
Practise using both the underside and the top of your tongue during oral sex. The underside will have a smoother feel as it lacks the bumpy papillae of the upper surface. Switch between the two surfaces to surprise and excite him.

an agile tongue
Practise pointing your tongue to work and strengthen the tip so the sensation it delivers is more defined. Stick your tongue out as far as you can and wiggle it from side to side and up and down. Then, move it back into your throat – do this a few times to increase your agility. And work the back of your tongue by moving it in circles at the back of your throat.

a flexible mouth
Open your mouth as wide as you can – use your fingers to stretch it. This not only helps lip strength, it keeps them supple, too. Drink through a straw and blow bubbles to strengthen your palate and lip muscles.

improve coordination
Practise holding a sweet or a spoon on your tongue. Hold your tongue outside of your mouth and lift it up and down trying to keep the sweet in place. Stick your tongue out as much as you can and then move it from side to side, trying to avoid touching your lips.

> ### try this!
> *Next time you brush your teeth, brush your tongue gently too. Or buy a tongue scraper to get rid of excess bacteria – and reduce the risk of bad breath that can be caused by a build-up of bacteria.*

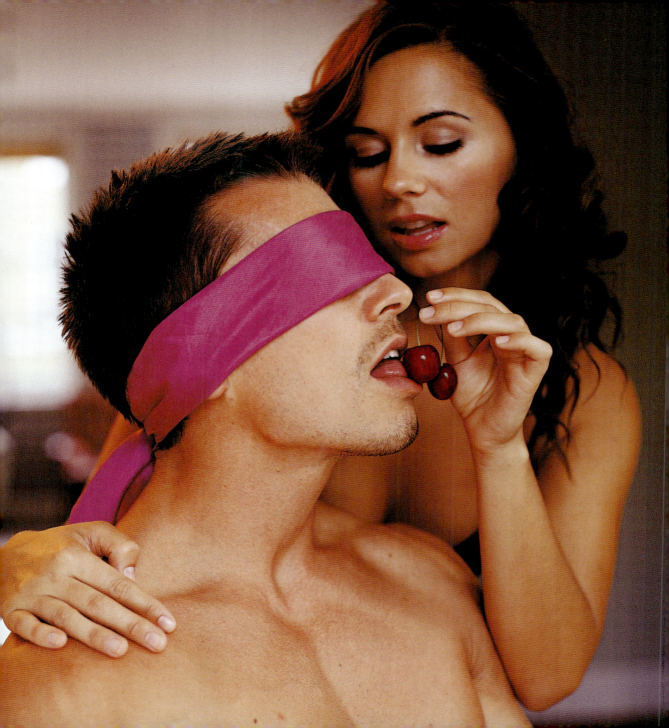

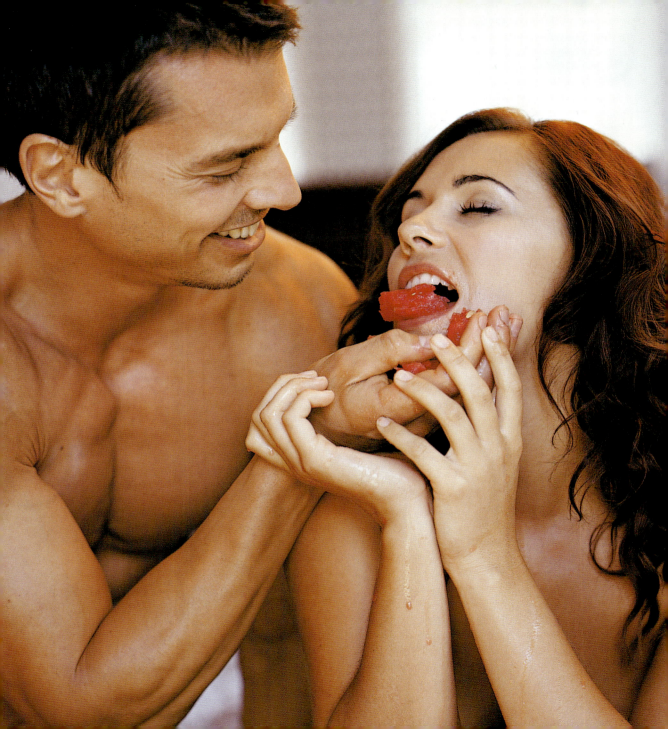

a warm playground

Try holding his flaccid penis in your mouth without tightening your lips around it, let it slide around – the sensation will feel exquisite for him and exciting for you because you will feel him grow bigger inside your mouth – very sexy. You can use the tip of your tongue to tickle his sweet spot – his frenulum – at the back of his glans.

try this!
If you're giving him a quickie here's a nifty trick to speed things up. Press the tip of your tongue into the roof of your mouth to promote saliva production. You will feel it pool underneath your tongue immediately.

what's in saliva?
Saliva is mostly water with mucus, chemicals and some antibacterial agents thrown in. It has several functions – it helps us to moisten and swallow food easily, coats the throat and it keeps our mouths clean and healthy and our breath fresh. It also helps to stop our teeth rotting.

Your salivary glands in your cheeks, mouth and jaw produce at least 2 pints of saliva a day. The amount produced varies according to hormonal changes in the body. A mouth full of saliva can make oral sex feel exquisite as it's a warm cushion for his penis.

a natural lubricant
Saliva is a natural lubricant for oral sex and handy because you never run out! Keep a glass of cold water nearby during oral sex to refresh yourself and stop your throat from drying out. By doing so, you will change the temperature of your mouth slightly and your partner will love it. Some men say that fellatio feels fantastic when their partner has a mouth full of saliva – the wetter the better! To him, your mouth feels like the inside of your vagina – wet, moist and slippery – but with the added benefits of allowing his penis free movement and more intense sensation.

lip-smackingly good

luscious lips

Your lips are there to help protect your mouth. The outside layer is dry skin, the inner lip mucousy — a mixture of rough and smooth, dry and wet that feels great to his penis. Yet, we often don't use all the parts of our lips when we're kissing or giving oral sex. A good kisser uses the inner lip as well as the outer lip to maximize sensation, friction and create moisture.

designed for kissing
Your lips are amazing — very muscular and strong yet also exquisitely sensitive and responsive to touch. The link between the lips and the clitoris in women is well reported, which is why kissing is such a turn-on because you can feel it in your groin. Who knows — it could be the same for men.

moisturize and colour
Soft, deliciously moist lips are a must for oral sex; dry, cracked ones simply won't do! Super-lips will make the whole experience much more sensual and erotic. Include your lips in your basic oral hygiene routine; exfoliate your lips by running a toothbrush over them gently. Add a little lip cream to moisturize before applying lipstick or lip gloss. It sounds like a cliché, but men are such visual creatures and the sight of your red, plump luscious lips wrapped around his cock will takes his breath away and stick in his mind — so that he remembers the blow job long after you've finished.

get your lips into shape
To exercise your puckering and pouting muscles, try out some whistling. Other ways of shaping up your lips include: filling your mouth with water and swirling it around a few times after teeth brushing; sucking hard on a piece of fruit and, the best is last, kissing with tongues every day — he won't complain, especially if you tell him it's to strengthen your lips for other activities!

> **try this!**
> Avoid any accidental nibbles by always wrapping your lips over your teeth during fellatio — unless he likes being nibbled, of course.

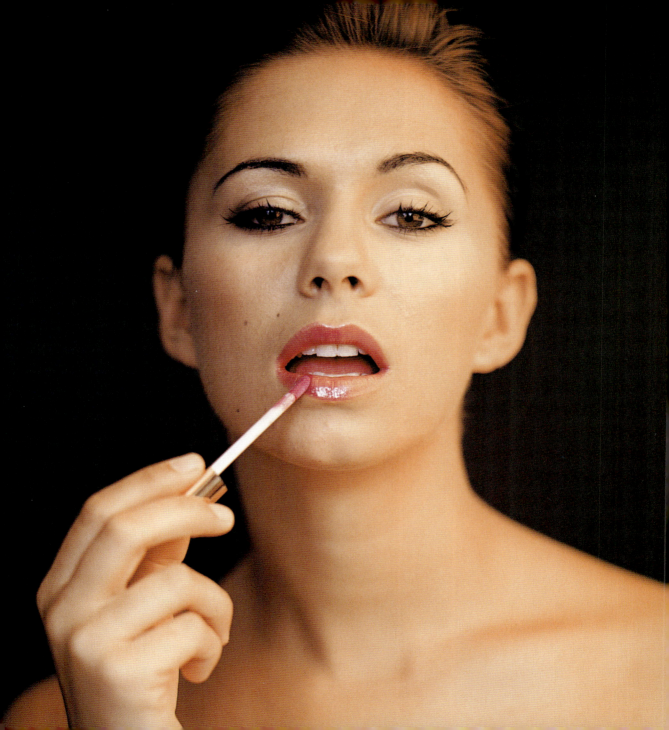

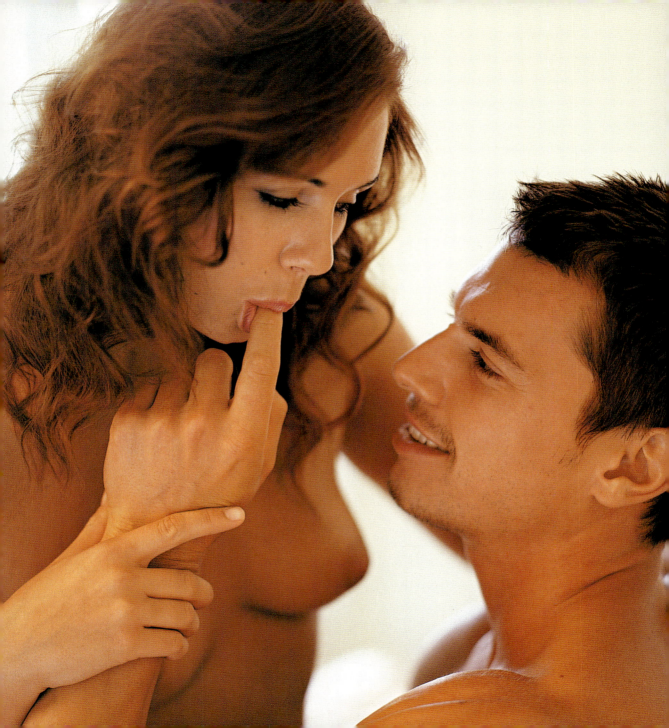

how's your jaw?

The U-shaped jaw bone (or mandible) joins your skull in front of your ears at the temporomandibular joint. Muscles attached to your jaw move this bone so that you can chew, bite and move your jaw from side to side. You'll find the junction beneath your ear where the lower jaw joins the skull: open your mouth widely until you can feel a soft space on your cheek with a finger.

common jaw complaints

Does your jaw give you problems or any pain? Common jaw complaints include clicking, slight pain when you bite into food and headaches. Causes include biting your nails and grinding your teeth in your sleep. Some people suffer with a lock jaw where the muscles tighten and they can't open their mouth very widely. Stress can also be a factor – you may be storing tension in your jaw and neck without realizing it. Regularly massage your jaw to overcome this. If you have a troublesome jaw long term, you won't be able to give your partner oral sex. Speak to your dentist if you're worried because it's usually not serious; or try the suggestions below first and visit the dental surgery if you're still bothered by it.

ask yourself...

If you have any jaw-related problem, try to isolate the possible cause. Ask yourself the following questions: Are you grinding your teeth or biting your nails? Are you stressed right now? Do you bite or nibble your lower lip? If you answer 'yes' to any, then read on for some help.

Avoid grinding your teeth or clenching your jaw – try to keep your face relaxed with the tip of your tongue at the top of your mouth. Relaxation is an important part of life, so make time to relax daily and have regular massages if you can afford it or learn a few self-massage techniques. If you need urgent attention, try using a hot-water bottle or hot towel wrapped around your neck/jaw to relieve the pain locally. And if your jaw hurts when you yawn, minimize the pain by lowering your head when you do so.

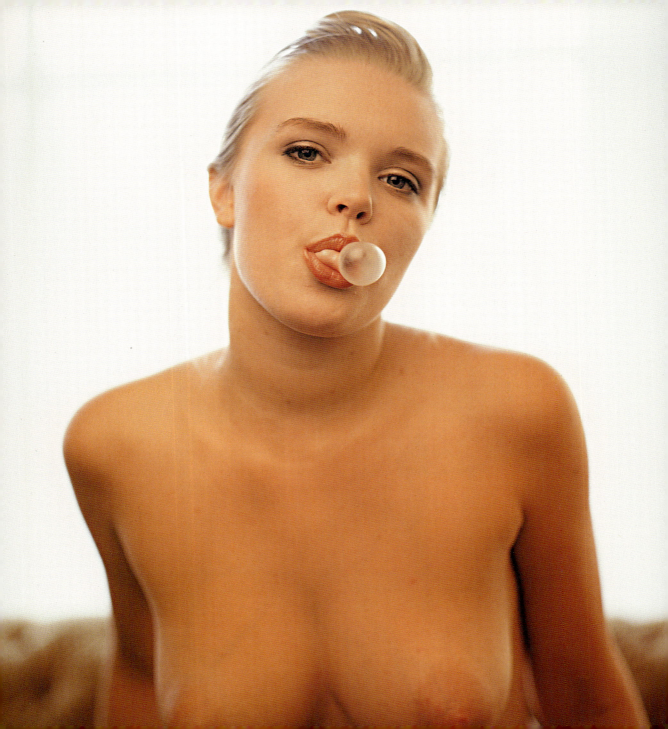

the jaw workout

Practise these jaw-strengthening exercises whenever you think about it for five minutes each time. As a bonus, these movements will help relax the muscles that work your jaw to keep it in tip-top shape.

> **try this!**
> Fill your mouth with crushed ice and then try to speak. This is a good starter for oral sex!

smoothly does it
Sit with a straight back for this one in a comfortable but upright chair. Keep your mouth closed and rest the tip of your tongue on the roof of your mouth. While keeping your teeth together, move the tip along the top palate until it reaches your tonsils. You should feel the muscle working – a slight pull in your lower jaw. Now, open your mouth slowly until your tongue moves away from the palate. Hold for a few seconds and relax. Ideally keep your movements slow and controlled.

circles in the air
Strengthen the neck and jaw area with this easy-to-do-anywhere exercise. Lower your chin to your chest and roll your neck from side to side slowly. Lift your neck and make circles.

gotta chew
Chew gum regularly because it creates saliva, keeps your teeth clean and breath fresh, and your throat well lubricated. It also gives your jaw muscles a workout.

enunciate your words
When you speak make sure you say words fully and properly – make a special effort with your vowels. It's very easy to become lazy with our words but you'll notice a big difference in the mobility of your mouth and lips if you make the effort with your speech. Try to get into the habit of using longer words to describe things in everyday conversations and also have fun with tongue twisters: Peter Piper Picked a Peck of Pickled Peppers (deep breath…).

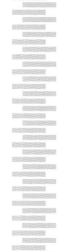

breath works best

Now that you're on your way to a super-fit mouth, tongue and jaw, turn your attention to your breathing to maximize the improvements so far. So, practise these exercises regularly to build strength in the right muscles – as well as relaxing you, they will help to improve your oral techniques.

singing in the rain
Well, sing in the shower at least – it helps you to breathe more consciously from your belly. Shallow breathing makes you feel anxious whereas deep breathing from the abdomen relaxes you. Studies have shown that singing also releases endorphins – your brain's feel-good chemicals – and puts you in a good mood.

breathe in and relax
Deep breathing lowers your blood pressure, relaxes muscles, counters stress and quells anxiety. Plus, it promotes better sleeping patterns. Practise this exercise for 15 minutes a day and you'll soon notice a huge difference in your mood. Lie down with your arms by your side. Put one hand on your tummy and feel your breath moving as it rises and falls. Try to breathe through your nose from your abdomen so it rises rather than your chest. Tense and relax each body part in turn, starting from your toes up to your head.

circular breathing
This exercise is often practised during meditation and is great for clearing the nasal passages, concentrating the mind and balancing the body. Sit with your knees crossed and back straight. Hold one finger over your left nostril and breathe in through the right. Hold once you've inhaled fully and slowly let the breath out again through the same nostril, keeping your finger in place. Repeat a few times on the same nostril then switch.

breath as a life force
Breathing is unconscious and mostly we breathe shallowly via our chest rather than deeply, via the abdomen. Breathing correctly boosts energy levels, vitality, creativity and blood circulation – in other words, it helps improve your sex life.

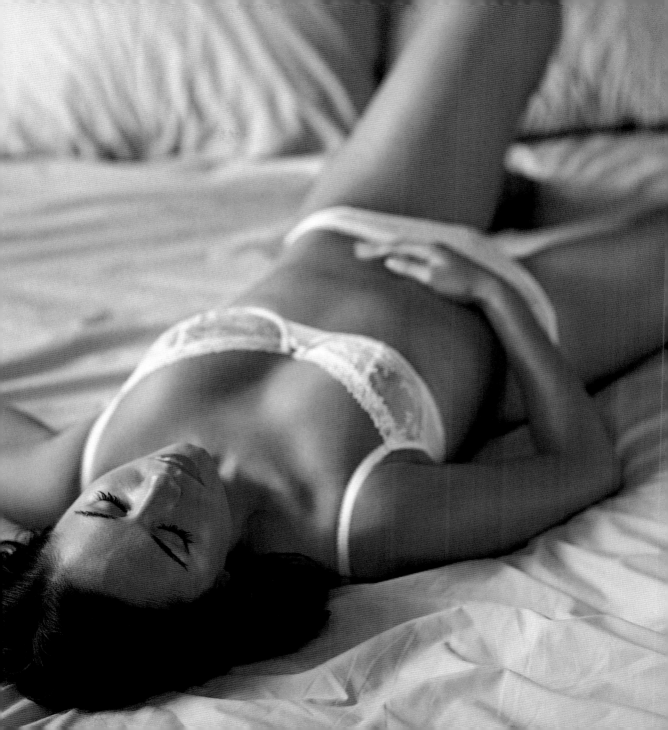

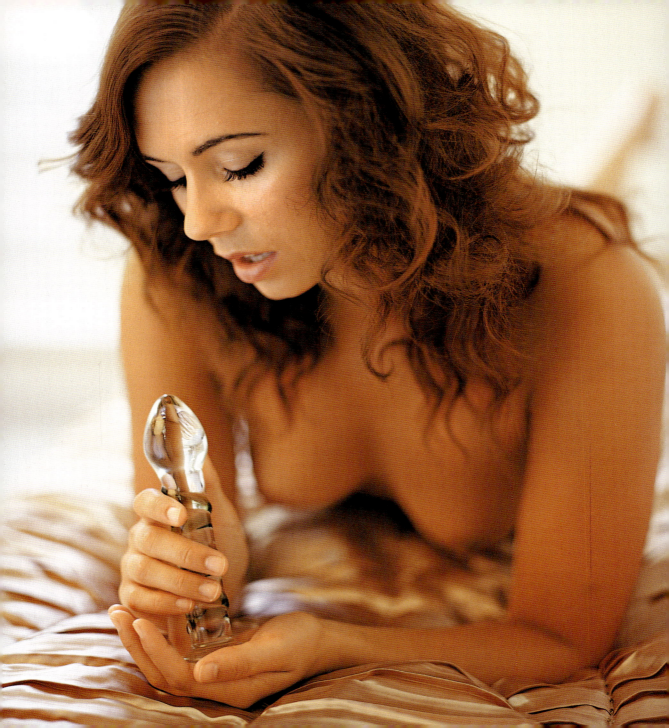

practice makes perfect

It's a good idea to practise before you give fellatio. It will increase your skill, improve your technique and boost your confidence, as well as giving you an idea of exactly how much and for how long you want him in your mouth.

try a dildo
Silicone dildos come in different sizes and are phallic in shape; you could even use one to practise deepthroating, if you wish. They don't smell or taste strange plus they won't break. Silicone also adjusts to your body's temperature so it is comfortable to use. Why not test out various flavoured lubricants, condoms and gels (always a good idea in case you hate the taste) while you're at it? The only difference between dildos and the real deal is the lack of response! Think of it as a patient penis. You could also try attaching a strap-on dildo to some furniture to free up your hands and make your practice session feel more realistic.

something a bit fruity
If you don't like the idea of a dildo, you could use any fruit or vegetables that are phallic in shape for some oral practice, but beware that cucumbers and zucchini may break mid-action, which could cause choking, especially if you're deepthroating. So, instead use root vegetables, which are sturdier, such as carrots, parsnips and potato. If they're not phallic, then you could have fun carving knob shapes out of them.

tongue twisting
Surprise your partner by learning how to put a condom on with your tongue; even practise on a dildo first or a phallic vegetable. This trick will get your tongue into serious shape as well as turning him on big time. If he's been complaining about using condoms then this is sure to change his mind.

Unroll the condom a little and put it into your mouth – teat first (unlubricated ones taste best). The other bit remains wrapped around your lips. Gently roll it down his penis, keeping your mouth pursed and slightly sucking as you go to ease it on. Now, use your hands to put it on fully.

the right angle
Lie back with your head off the edge of the bed to practise deepthroating. The angle of your neck helps your throat to open up so that you can take the dildo (or him) deeper.

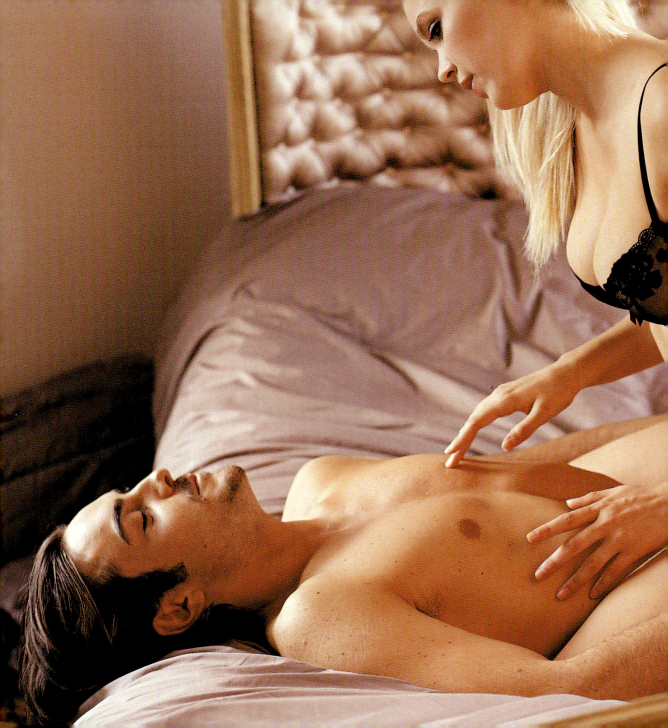

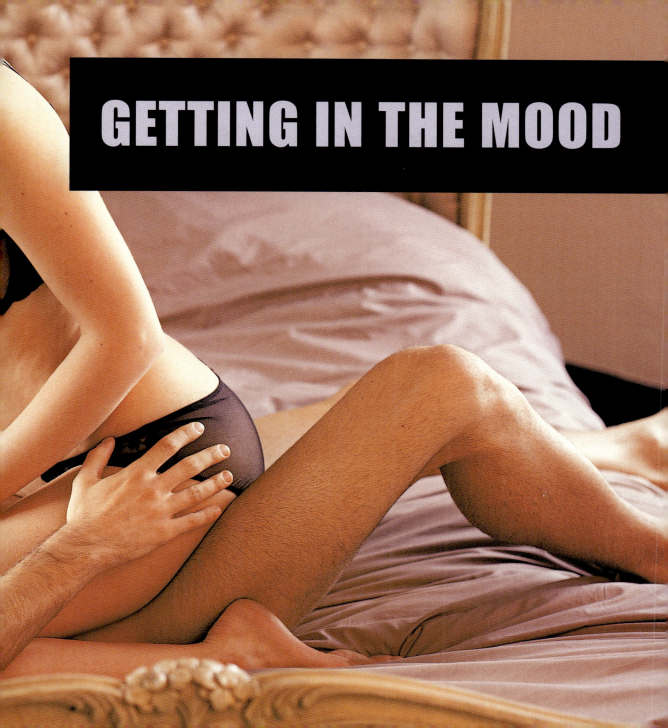

GETTING IN THE MOOD

This chapter covers foreplay – the essential ingredient for successful fellatio. The best sex incorporates a lot of foreplay and he will enjoy the tease and anticipation as much as you do. Do it well for him and you'll give him plenty of ideas so he can reciprocate. Foreplay is everything from kissing and cuddling to erotic massage and feasting; to bathing together and sharing fantasies. This intimate contact will keep each other's motors running during the day – so that when you get home you're racing to the bedroom. It keeps the spirit of your relationship alive.

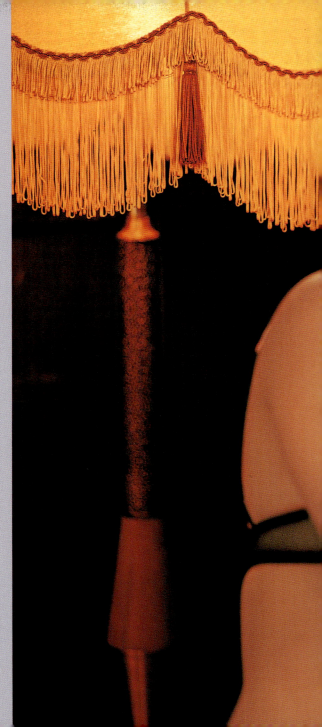

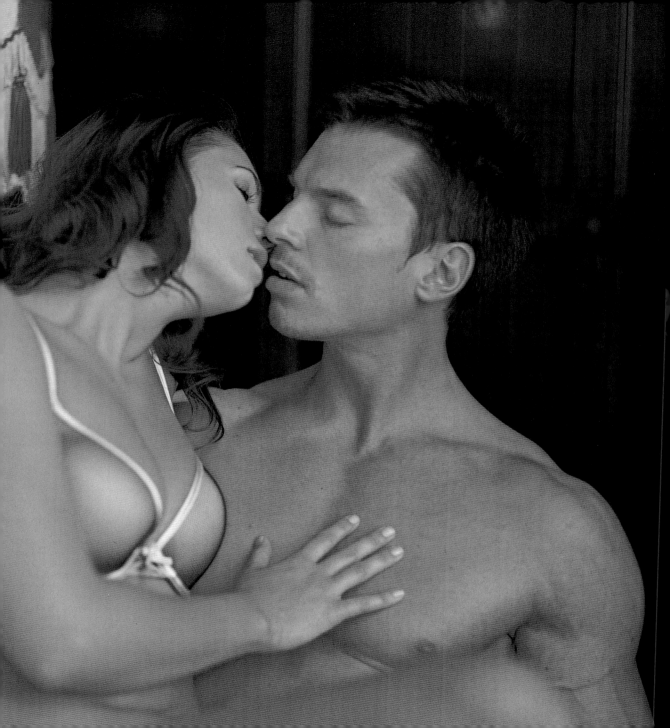

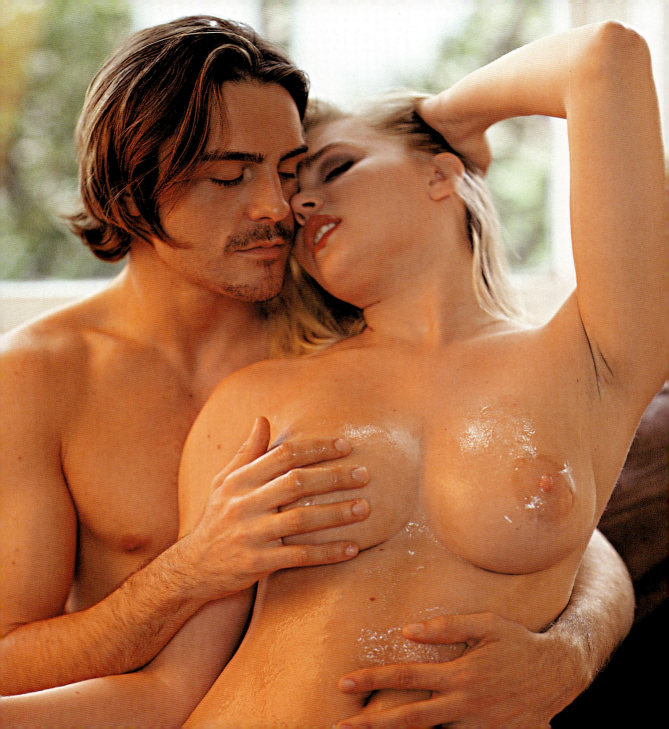

foreplay

You know the drill – low lighting, candles, music to grind to, sensual fabrics and smells. You're engaging each sense, providing some kind of stimulation so that you're both in the moment and fully in your bodies. Foreplay engages your brain and your imagination, and gets your sexual energies moving in sync so that oral sex is more fulfilling and exciting for you both.

what is foreplay?

Foreplay is: about being creative, spontaneous and relaxed. Understanding your partner and making personal touches, reading his body language and making him feel good about himself and desired.

Foreplay isn't: about spending large amounts of money on sexy lingerie or hotels or wearing (or doing) something that makes you feel uneasy or uncomfortable.

getting naked

Being naked strips you to your core and helps to break down any communication barriers. It brings you back to basics – being in the moment and experiencing pleasure through your bodies and senses. It's your natural state of being and one that too often gets forgotten. If you feel comfortable in your body then that's a whole lot sexier than being dressed in something for the sake of 'sexiness'.

bathing together

This essential part of your relaxation routine gives you both time to unwind from your day. How often do you wash each other all over? Shampoo each other's hair and sponge and wash your bodies. Lather up your hands and wash his genitals for him (and rinse well) – especially important if you're hoping to pleasure him orally later. Shaving each other's genitals can also be very sexy and intimate, and it can vastly improve oral sex (see page 74).

toy box

Have your box of tricks (toys, lube) handy so that you aren't running around looking for things once you've started. Keep it by the bed.

smooch

Kissing is a hugely important part of foreplay. Weave your way around his body paying attention to all his hot spots – his neck and nipples, and his inner thighs – before you get to his genitals. Create the anticipation for what's to come – when he discovers that your mouth feels just as good (if not better) than your vagina. Slip your fingers into his mouth and ask him to suck and kiss them the way he'd like you to fellate him. Kissing sets the scene for what's to come next.

cuddling

According to the Taoists cuddling helps to harmonize our bodies. You can do this effectively by lying on top of your partner or vice versa and aligning your body parts – hands, lips, genitals, feet and so on – for at least 10 minutes. This position will help you to build your sexual tension. Oral sex moves one step on from this – you are putting opposite body parts together – your mouth to his genitals, for example, to 'stir' sexual energy.

fantasies

Share erotic fantasies with each other. Does he have a fantasy about where or how he'd like to receive oral sex? And, do you? Write your fantasies on pieces of paper and put them into a hat. Choose one to perform each week.

give porn a go

Experiment with different types of porn – this will give you more oral tips and techniques. Porn is pretty creative these days and there's something for everyone – lesbian porn will give you a few ideas about how to fellate a strap-on cock.

sexy sounds

Choose your music – heavy rock if that works for you or mellow chilled-out grooves if that's more your kind of thing. You need to be able to lose yourself in the music. And, absolutely, turn off your mobile phone; don't ever be tempted to stop mid-way to take a phone call. It's a sure-fire passion killer!

dressing the part

Choose an outfit you feel sexy in, paint your nails and lips to make oral sex a more visual treat for him. Nice nails are a must. If your hair is long, tie it up so he can see the expressions on your face and you can maintain eye contact during the act. Experiment with your clothes once in a while and try out different fabrics to make oral sex feel more sensual – he can feel your knickers on his thighs when you straddle him – so make sure they are silky. If you fancy a change, you could try leather, rubber or PVC, but keep in mind that comfort and flexibility are key (see also page 122).

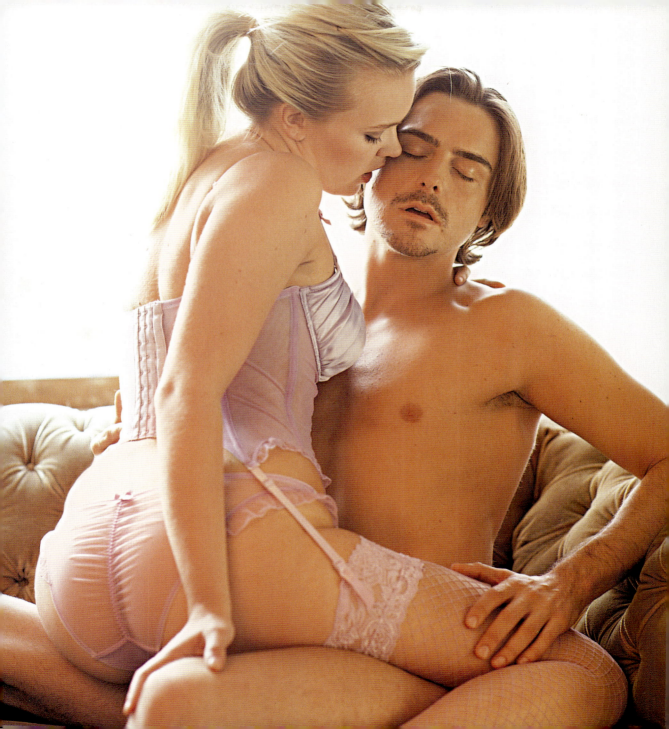

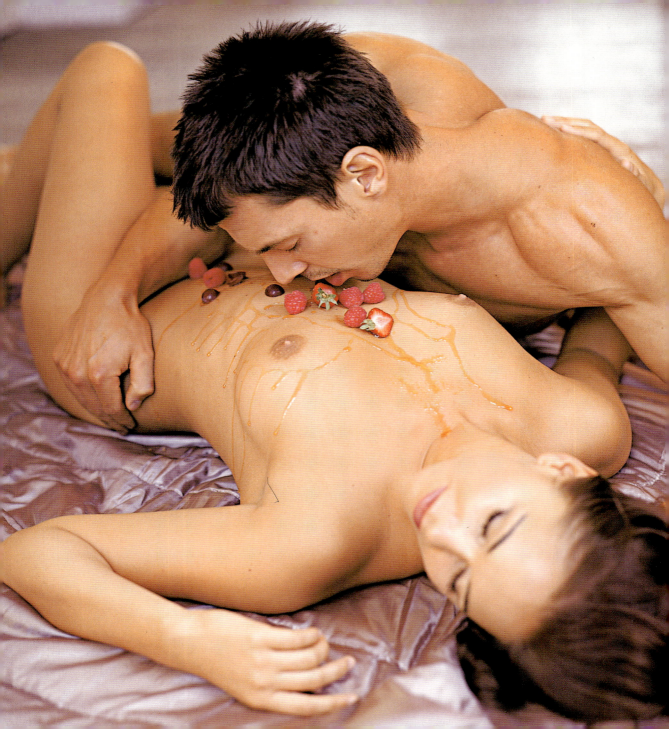

a feast for two

It's fun to experiment with different tastes, smells and textures to awaken your palate and senses. Seek out sensual foods to increase your sexual pleasure – it's great foreplay for you both. Eating well puts you in a good mood, keeps you in the moment and will prepare your mind and body for a sexual feast.

aphrodisiac foods

Food and sex are strongly linked in mythology. The term 'aphrodisiac' comes from the Greek goddess for sensuality, Aphrodite. Ancient civilizations used to enjoy feasting before sex and appreciated the power of food to enhance wellbeing and libido. They believed that foods that resembled the genitals, such as figs, oysters, peaches and apples, or those that came from a seed, bulb or root had special powers to enhance sexuality and so made a habit of eating them!

feeling fruity?

Certain foods can sweeten the taste of semen making oral sex nicer for you if you want to swallow his come. Feed him fruits at breakfast or have him eat them off your body using only his mouth. Get him to dribble honey over your breasts and tummy to fix the berries in place for a visual treat before he feasts. Good fruits to use are strawberries, raspberries, lychees, melon, pineapple, mangoes, apples, cherries and kiwi.

keep him sweet

Chocolate contains a natural 'love drug' phenylethylamine (a natural chemical that we release when we're in love), which stimulates the brain's pleasure centres and reaches peak levels during orgasm. Plus, chocolate also contains tryptophan, which the brain uses to make serotonin – another 'feel good' chemical. Share it in bed and melt some down (cool it a little first) to dribble on his body during oral sex and lick off.

body sushi

Nyotaimori is the Japanese practice of eating raw fish off a naked woman's body. Recreate your own table dining at home – make some sushi and finger foods, such as cream cheese on cucumber, raw vegetables and rolls of thin ham. Lay them on his naked body, tell him to lie very still and eat slowly using your mouth only.

erotic shaving

Shaving each other 'down below' can massively improve oral sex. It looks hot – you can see each other's genitals and watch what happens when he gets excited (and yes, it makes his penis look bigger). It feels wonderful – soft and silky, free and open, and it will make your bodies slide and glide. What's more, it's an intimate act of trust that can bring you closer.

your shaving kit

Wet shaving is more intimate and sexier than dry shaving. You'll need a decent razor – two- or three-bladed are fine; and use a fresh blade each time. Choose one that feels nice to hold and looks good too, as the tools are part of the experience. Choose a good-quality shaving cream or oil (foam can irritate his pores) and a shaving brush (badger hair is best) to exfoliate the skin at the same time.

secrets of successful shaving

Trim the pubic hairs using nail scissors until it's short enough to shave. Decide where exactly you're going to shave – he may not want to shave the whole genital area. Then, take a bath together – warm water opens the pores and makes the skin easier to shave.

Pull the skin taut and take it slowly; always shave in the direction of the hair growth to reduce irritation. Once you've shaved, do it again sideways to get a closer shave. Don't panic if you see bumps, spots or rashes the first time around – the skin needs time to adjust.

down to the shaving

Pull the skin on his penis taut and shave in a downward direction – don't do it more than twice on the same spot as it can cause razor rash. Hold the base and shave down the shaft in one stroke until you've covered the lot. Next do his inner thighs – another sensitive area so it will feel quite sexy to him. It's easier to do his scrotum if he's turned on, so ask him to masturbate a little beforehand or try nipple clamps. A smooth, hair-free anus is a must for oral sex. Get him to bend over, gently spread his cheeks and lightly shave the area. Finish off with a rinse in cool water to tighten the skin and apply some moisturizing cream to prevent razor rash.

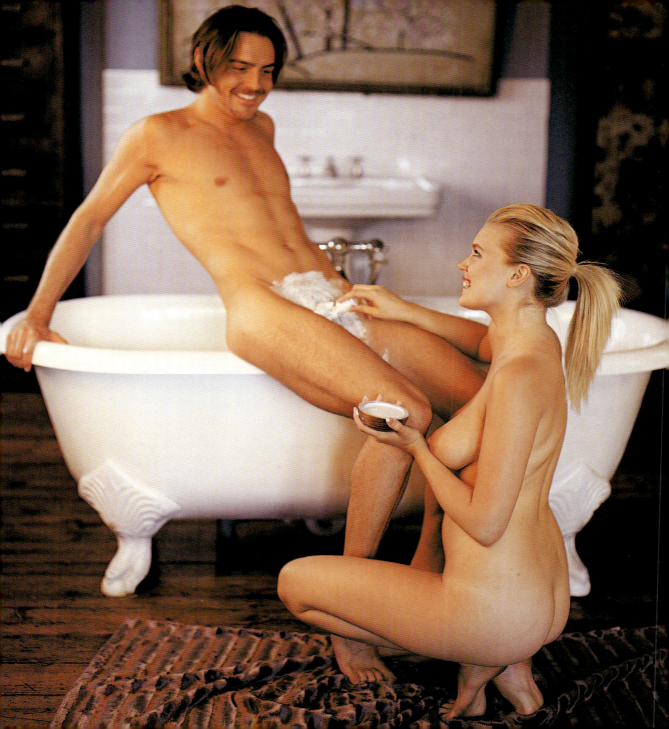

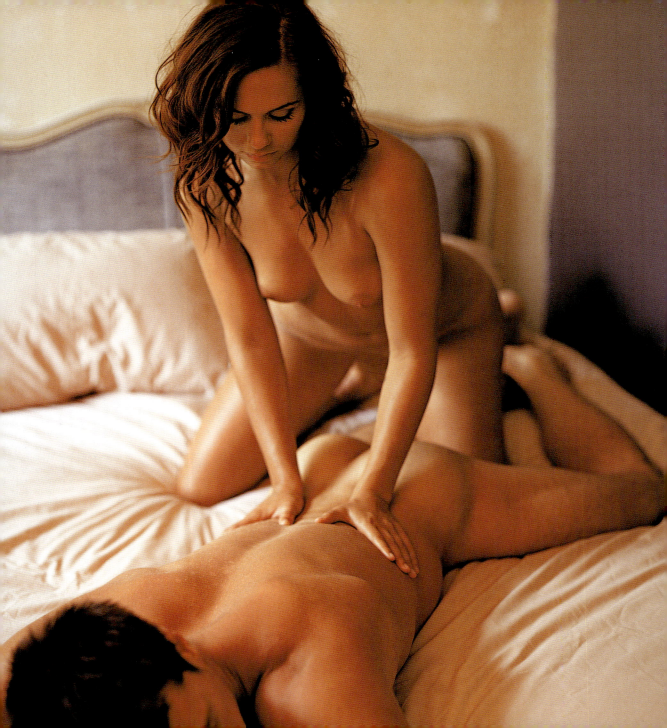

erotic massage

Massage is a great primer for oral sex. It relaxes both of you, keeps you 'in the moment' and puts you in a good mood. What's more, it can boost your sexual energy. Technique-wise, use the pad of your finger not the fingertip (or your knuckle) and apply varying levels of pressure, hold for 10–15 seconds and then release and repeat.

arousing acupressure

Certain acupressure points on your body are linked to your genitals – your sexual core. Massaging these areas can help to shift energy blocks and boost libido. You can think of your body in terms of 14 energy meridians – six on each half of your body and another two running down the centre at the front and back. They work in pairs – one being yin (the feminine energy) and the other yang or masculine energy.

relaxing reflexology

Various reflexology points on the foot can give both libido and sexual energy a lift when pressure is applied to them. Giving each other a foot massage before oral sex can help you both unwind.

acupressure points

These acupressure points turn up the heat in terms of your sexual energy:

Gv4 *– between the second and third vertebrae along your spine. This stimulates the kidneys, which are thought to affect your sexual energy if low.*

B47 *– a hand's width from your spine, near the second and third vertebrae.*

B23 *– base of the spine/sacral area.*

Sp6 *– just above the ankle bone on the inside of your leg.*

Cv4/6 *– middle of the tummy below your navel and can help with impotence.*

Li8 *– inner side of the knee.*

St36 *– just below the knee on the front of the leg and helps balance testosterone.*

It gets rid of tension in the body, and you can use it as a signal for your mutual relaxation time. The main area to concentrate on, however, is the heel of the foot and around the anklebone – this is where the genital points are primarily located.

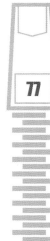

lingam massage

According to Taoists the penis is packed with reflexology points – far more so than the hands or the feet – that correspond to parts of the body. They believe that there is a direct connection between the genitals and the internal organs. So, go Taoist for the day and massage his cock before indulging in oral sex.

penis reflexology
Pleasure him by applying pressure to the penis' reflexology points to allow him to surrender to so-called 'organ' orgasms, which last for up to 10 hours or more. But, bear in mind, the goal is to massage but *not* to bring him to orgasm.

his 'wand of light'
Once you've made your partner comfortable, ask him to lie back and relax. Ensure your hands are well lubricated and start by massaging his shaft – it doesn't matter if his erection comes and goes. Hold him at the base and alternate one hand on top of the other – moving them up and down in a rhythm. Imagine that you are unscrewing a bottle or squeezing an orange and keep it continuous.

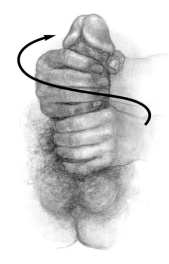

Find his frenulum – on the back of the glans – and manipulate it gently between your thumbs. If he looks as if he's going to come, back off and encourage him to breathe deeply. Now, push the shaft back so it reaches towards his tummy. You can tickle his underbelly (men love this) and this will help circulate the sexual energy in the rest of his body. When you've finished, cup his penis and hold for a few seconds as a signal of the end. Now, gently remove your hands, cover him and keep him warm. Allow him to rest for 5–10 minutes.

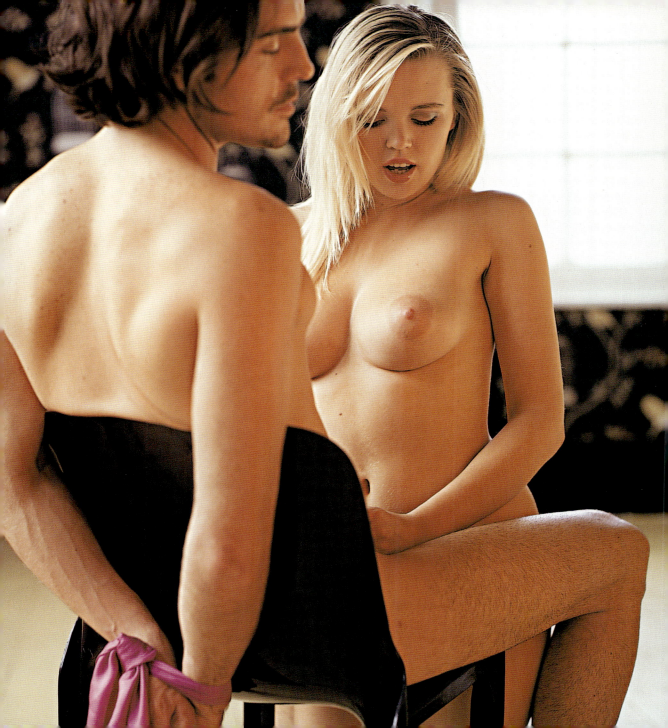

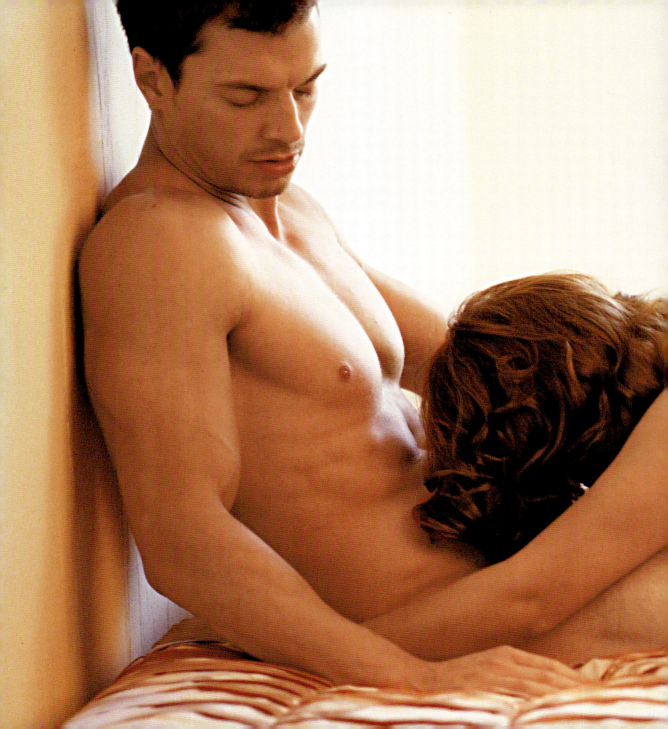

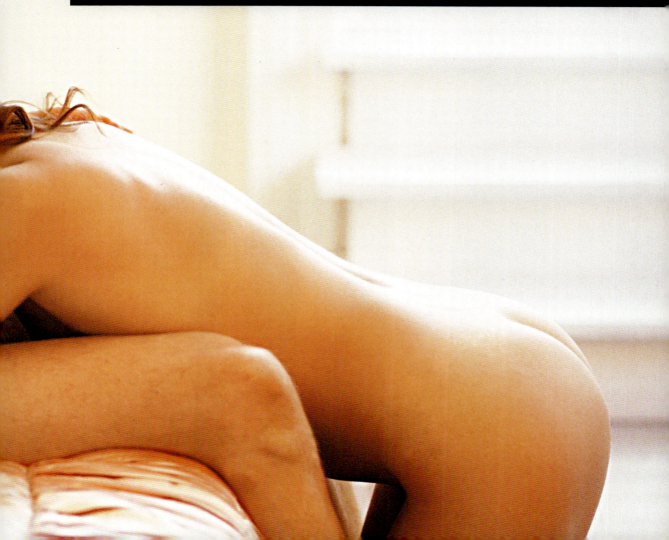

Most of us enjoy oral sex but when asked which position we like to do it in there are a few puzzled looks. Positions for oral sex? Doesn't that come afterwards with intercourse? Well, it's time to shake things up a little. There are many positions for fellatio and you might find that some feel better than others because of the angle of the penis in your mouth. It's also sexy and fun to try new things – be creative with each other and experiment.

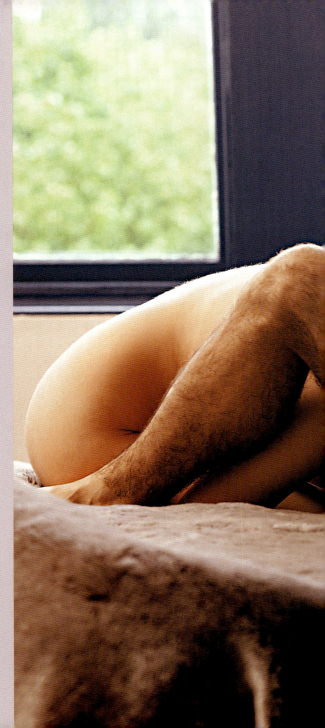

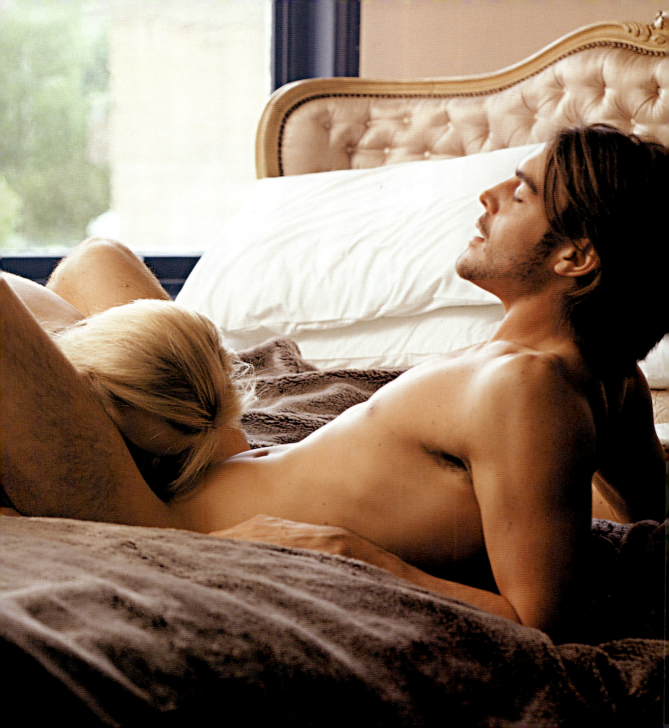

tricks of the trade

Once you've found a position and technique that works for you both it's tempting to use it every time. The problem is that when we become too familiar we lose interest and our bodies stop responding in the same way. Giving oral sex in the same way, time after time will become boring for you both. So, every now and then mix things up a bit.

suck, kiss, lick and 'blow'

There are many ways of kissing so learn a few new ones: soft, hard, nibbling, biting, sucking. Kiss him all over – everywhere. Then, start licking his shaft from bottom to top (to give him a sense of his length). If he likes it, nibble the shaft gently and drag it gently back up with your teeth. Suction-wise, you don't want to go too hard.

Blow gently on the glans and the length of the shaft after you've licked it. Next, practise 'tea bagging' where you take one ball into your mouth and suck it; most men love this. If when you're sucking the glans you try to swallow at the same time, the movements will pull his penis back into your throat creating intensely pleasurable sensations, which he'll love.

temperature's rising

Now you know where his perineum, prostate gland and million-dollar point are, heighten his pleasure by stimulating them. And since moisture lessens friction keep things wet (with saliva or lubricant) for gliding movements and superb sensations. Breathe in as you come up his shaft and then exhale as you go down – it will feel cool on the way up and hotter back down. Add extra spice by popping some alcohol or ice in your mouth just before taking him in.

mix it up

Vary your technique – use your hands at the same time or to give your mouth a break. Go down lightly and up firmly – then switch. When he's close to orgasm keep the rhythm steady and continuous to drive him over the edge. And, hold his knees down when he comes – for a more intense orgasm that stays concentrated in his genitals.

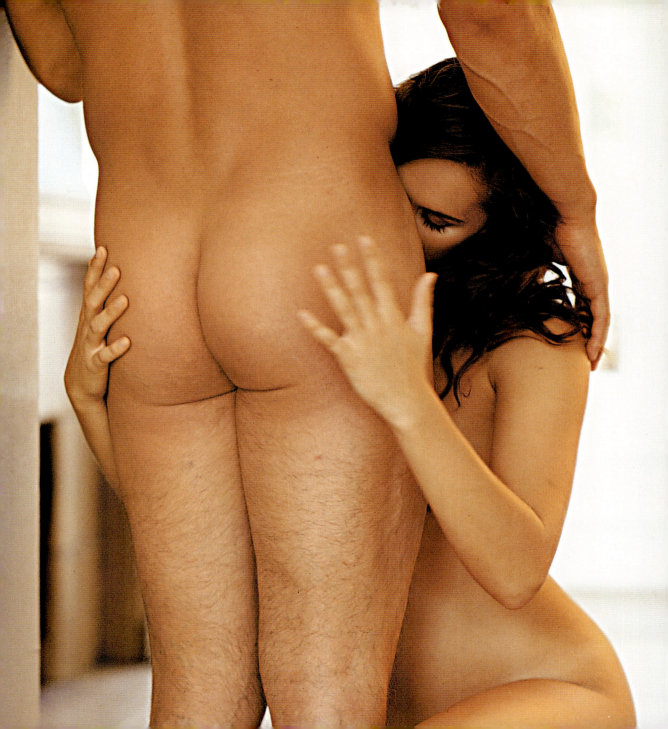

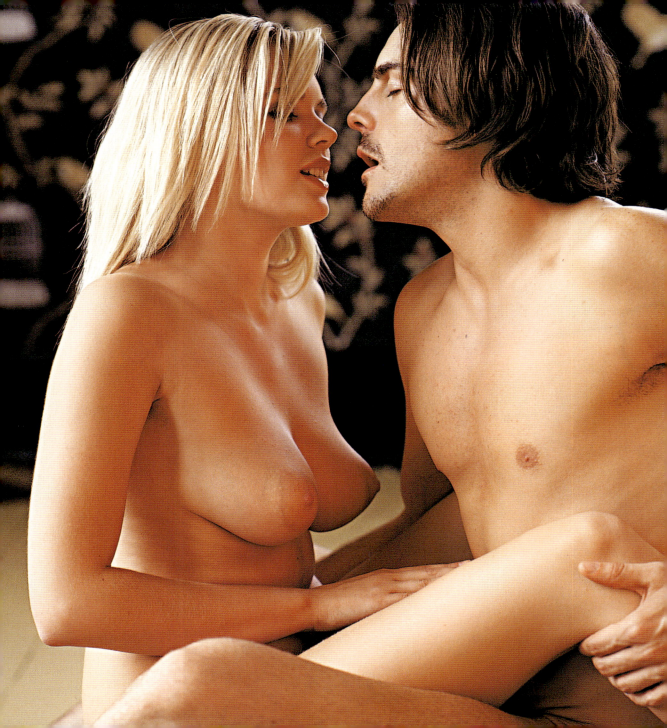

hand tricks

Give your mouth a break or use these techniques to start off your oral sex session. Watch your man to monitor how he's enjoying what you're doing. If he's in seventh heaven, his legs will relax and open a little wider, he'll moan, his skin will flush and his breathing will get heavier. And you'll know when he's about to come as a small amount of pre-ejaculate appears on his glans.

squeeze and hold
Hold his penis firmly at the base in one hand, forming a ring around it. Move your other hand up and down his shaft, squeezing your hands along it rhythmically until you reach the tip. This quick and easy penis massage stimulates his other body parts as mentioned (see page 78). This squeeze and hold technique will energize his entire body.

circle dance
Form your finger and thumb into a circle and dance it up and down his cock. It's best to use plenty of lube so that the smooth fluid movement replicates the sensation of entering your vagina. Pay attention to the glans and keep the circle fairly tight, especially when moving off and back on to it, to maximize his sensations.

body clock
Are your hands warm? If not, then rub them together to warm them up and plop some lube in the palms. Keeping one palm flat, rhythmically rub it across the top of the glans, making circles in one direction. Now, change direction. As his glans is exquisitely sensitive, massaging here will bring him to the brink and push him over the edge into an explosive orgasm in no time at all.

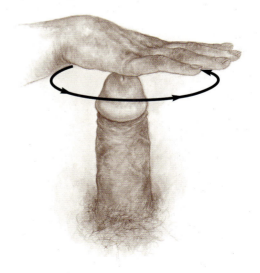

underbelly

The underside of the penis is also incredibly sensitive but is often ignored. See if your man likes a bit of action here. Push his penis on to his stomach to expose it, and then gently massage from bottom to top, using lots of lubricant for smooth sliding movements. Work out if he's got a super-hot spot – many men do – on the underside of his penis and concentrate on it once you've found it. Cup his testicles and scrotum in warm hands, too – he'll love you for it.

lacing

Lace your fingers together keeping them as straight as you can. Cup his penis between your palms and fingers, and work him into a frenzy. Use some lube to maximize the sensation. And if he's standing, why not spank his buttocks to get the endorphins racing and make his climax stronger and harder?

the pump

Once you've mastered the lacing technique, turn up the heat a notch. This time lace your fingers but clasp your fingers together so they are curved over one another rather than straight. Hold and pump him up and down from the base to the top and back down again. Keep movements smooth with lots of lube and change direction to keep him on his toes.

> **try this!**
>
> *Mix things up a bit by varying the pressure and stroke to keep him guessing what's going to happen next.*
>
> - *Alternate between a light and firm grip, squeeze and slide, rub and stroke his cock to vary it. Stretch the skin to maximize sensation. Use your thumbs, fingers and the front and back of your hands.*
> - *Pay attention to his crown jewels – testicles and scrotum.*
> - *Warm him up slowly by massaging his shaft and ignoring his glans – watch it grow bigger as he gets more excited.*

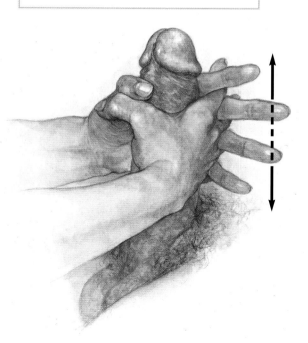

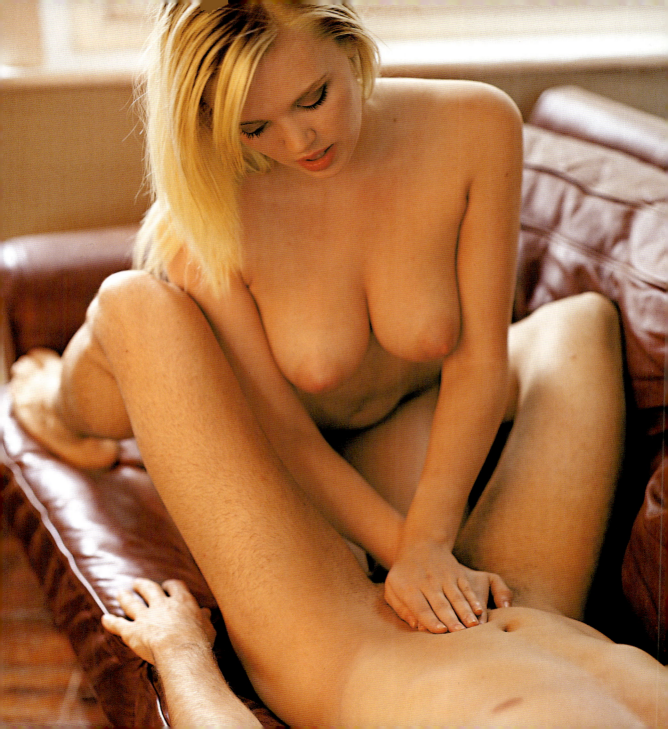

hand and mouth combos

The secret to giving a great blow job is in using your hands at the same time – so that he can't tell the difference. That said, think of fellatio as something you do with your whole body. Play up to it a little: work your body; raise your buttocks; play with your breasts; let him see you enjoying yourself and feeling sexy. Maintain eye contact with him and learn how to tell if he's really enjoying himself so you'll know instinctively what's working for him and what isn't.

prick tease

Don't be afraid to stop and start to build tension and excitement – it's a blow job not a rush job, after all. Start off by running your hands up and down the shaft, and massage everywhere but the glans. Ignore it. As you do so, it will enlarge and darken in colour as he becomes more excited. Play with his balls and carry on massaging the shaft. When he's moaning for more, surprise him by licking the glans. Now, hold it in your mouth or massage it to bring him to climax. His orgasm, when it comes, will be much more intense and you will feel immensely powerful.

slow dance

With your partner on his back, bend over him – or vice versa. Prolong the tease and allow his orgasm to build, put his penis in your mouth and keep your lips open so that he's sliding in and out of your mouth. Pull his legs apart to prolong the excitement and hold his testicles away from his body as he nears orgasm – delaying things a little will intensify his orgasm.

quick step

If you fancy a 'quickie' then lick along the underbelly of his penis from bottom to top, focusing on the glans when you get there. Do this several times quickly and then suck on the glans intensely keeping a rhythm all the time. He will come fast and furious. Why not push him further and stimulate his prostate at the same time?

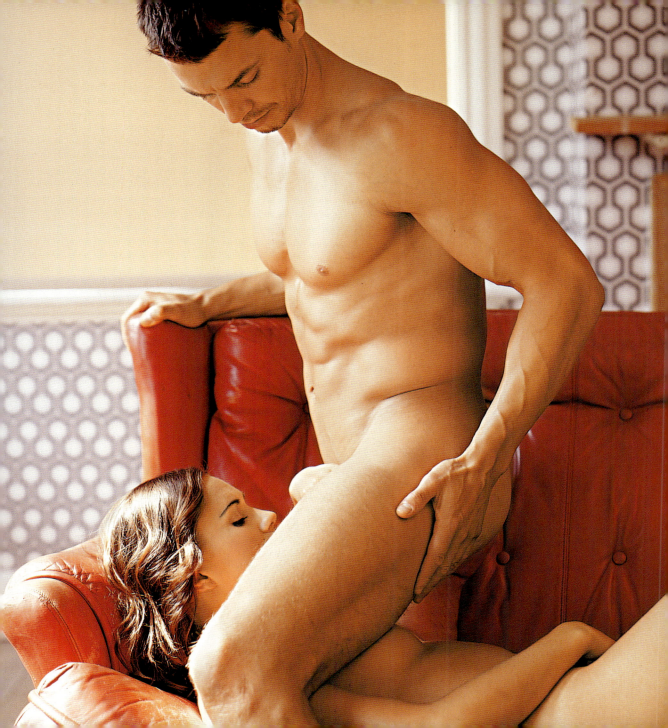

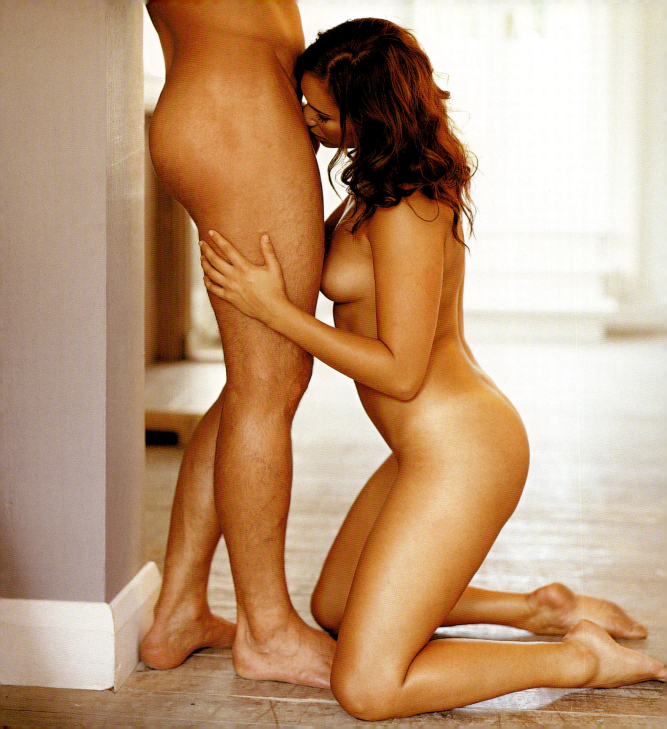

the warrior

This fantastic starter position for oral sex gives you the freedom to slip into other poses easily, especially if you want to have full-on sex afterwards. Standing positions like this one are great for quickies because they're impulsive and you can take him by surprise, so take your man by the hand and lead him anywhere you fancy – outdoors, around the house, even in the office – and he could be fully clothed or half-dressed if needs must.

fancy a quickie?

Grasp your spontaneity by the balls and initiate oral sex in this active position your man will adore. Lean him against the wall and kneel down to centre yourself between his legs, with your knees slightly apart. Reach round his thighs and hold on to give yourself some support.

Once you've taken him by surprise, practise unzipping his trousers with your teeth! When you take hold of his cock, create a ring with your fingers around its base to control how deep and fast he thrusts, because he's sure to want to pump away.

why not...?

Keep him guessing by tying his hands behind his back and blindfolding him so he can't predict your moves. Or, if you prefer, position him where there is a big mirror behind you so he can watch your every move – and you, of course – from the rear.

Remember to pay attention to all his hot spots – scrotum, balls, buttocks, anus and inner thighs; and why not have a break and play with yourself or let him caress your breasts, hair and face?

Because you're working with gravity, this upright pose can help keep his erection for longer. And, what's more, will give both of you an energetic workout.

Take it in turns – let him give you cunnilingus standing next time and you'll soon both have legs – and buttocks – of steel. If the inevitable happens and it turns into a longer session, manoeuvre him on to the bed so you're both more comfortable.

a perfect blow job every time

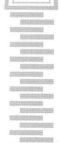

face-sitting

Your man is bound to love this active, dominant position where he feels as if he's in control – except it's you really directing the sex play. He'll be able to thrust and go deep if you want him to, plus he can watch exactly what you are doing, which is incredibly hot.

power play

Face-sitting can be a fun part of sex or power play. It can be a fantasy – the idea of being dominant and using your full body weight to sit over your partner and the fact that you are 'forcing' your partner to give you oral sex can intensify the experience for you both.

take him deep and hard

Lie back and get your partner to kneel over your face. Take his penis into your mouth and grasp his buttocks. Men often love this position as they can thrust deeply into your mouth and set the pace, so it feels doubly exciting for him. To control his thrusting, grip the base of his penis with your hands. He will still feel like he's in deep as he won't know where your mouth ends and your hands begin. This position makes deep thrusting easier as the angle of your throat is aligned with his penis.

why not...?

Turn him around so that he's crouched facing your feet and perform analingus. Tease, slap, rub and massage his buttocks first to warm him up and get the endorphins flowing. Then, gently spread his cheeks and rim him from top to bottom (it's wise to use a dental dam), increasing the pressure as you go. If you want, slip inside his anus as he gets more turned on. Reach between his legs to massage his penis, scrotum and testicles at the same time for a deeper orgasm.

sitting comfortably?

If this position strains your neck or your man's legs tire, then explore the world of erotic furniture. There are lots of really creative pieces out there, which can make sex a real giggle. Specially designed stools and chairs are available – he sits astride with his genitals through a hole in the middle. Using such props means that he's suspended over your face and his weight's supported, so you have room to move and he won't topple on to you mid-act!

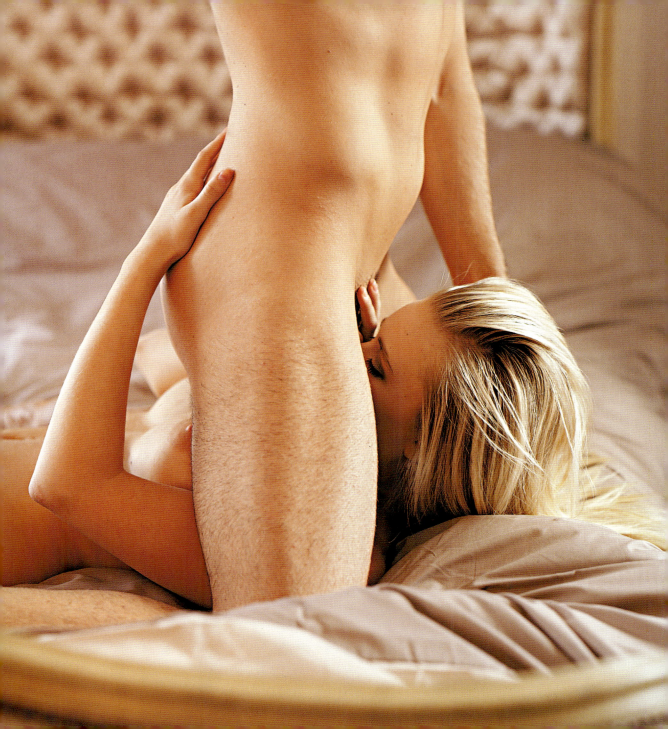

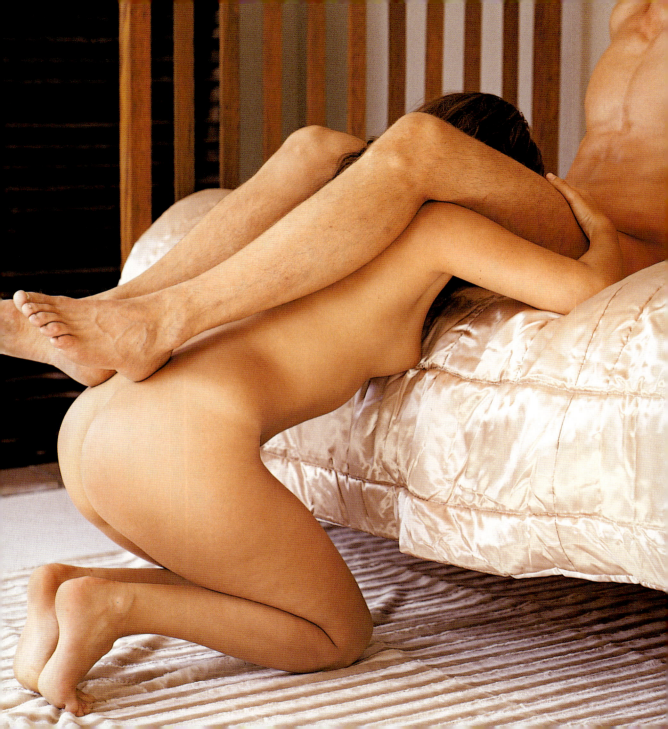

shoulder stand

The Japanese have a philosophy called 'kaizen', which means making small changes every day to change for the better. Apply this philosophy to your sex life by having oral sex at different times of the day or trying out new positions, such as this one. This unusual and fun position will give you both a giggle, if only because it feels a bit like you're in a yoga class.

why not...?
Switch positions if you need to keep him higher and your bed mattress is too soft; or use some pillows to raise him up a little. Alternatively, have a go with his legs over the edge of the sofa or a chair – just choose one that's at the right height and feels comfortable for you.

get down and dirty
With your partner lying on the edge of the bed, get him to drape his thighs over your shoulders. In this position, you can grip his thighs and fellate him while you're kneeling on the floor. Start by teasing him – nibbling and kissing your way up his inner thighs and caressing his scrotum, testicles and perineum before you reach his penis. If you get him to tilt his pelvis, you can reach and squeeze his buttocks and finger his anus.

It's a very relaxing position for your partner as he can lie back and do nothing but enjoy how it feels. If he wants to be more involved, however, he can prop a pillow behind his neck and lean forward for a closer view – or to fondle you.

It's a good idea to keep this session short and sweet, as his weight may put stress on your neck and shoulders. If you feel uncomfortable, then push him back on to the bed and straddle him instead.

sixty-nine

If you're looking for something fun and erotic you can do to turn each other on, then look no further. The 69 (or soixante-neuf) is a classic sex position that allows you to give each other oral sex at the same time. Because you're approaching each other's genitals from the opposite direction the sensation will differ so it's worth experimenting with. It's incredibly sexy to intertwine your bodies like this. And if your man's feeling strong, you can try out the variation opposite.

side-by-side or one on top?

With your partner lying down, straddle him first and then lie on top of him so that you face his feet. While he lies underneath you, he'll be able to push some of your buttons. Some people enjoy 69 and others think it's overrated. But it's well worth a try, even if you do lose your concentration when he does something fabulous. In fellatio, it works better if you're on top as you most probably weigh less.

why not...?

Try this position for a quickie if your man is feeling strong and energetic, and you are much lighter than him. He stands or crouches while holding you upside down, so that your head is between his legs. As your genitals will be at his head height he can bury his head and pleasure you at the same time. Standing feels good and it's a very masculine, active position.

If the on-top version isn't comfortable because of weight differences or mismatched height, then try lying side-by-side using pillows to keep your head and neck level to his genital area. This gives you both access to each other's hot spots and room to move freely so it feels more comfortable. Give your mouths a break every now and then and use your hands – you can also reach his buttocks and anal area fairly easily in this position.

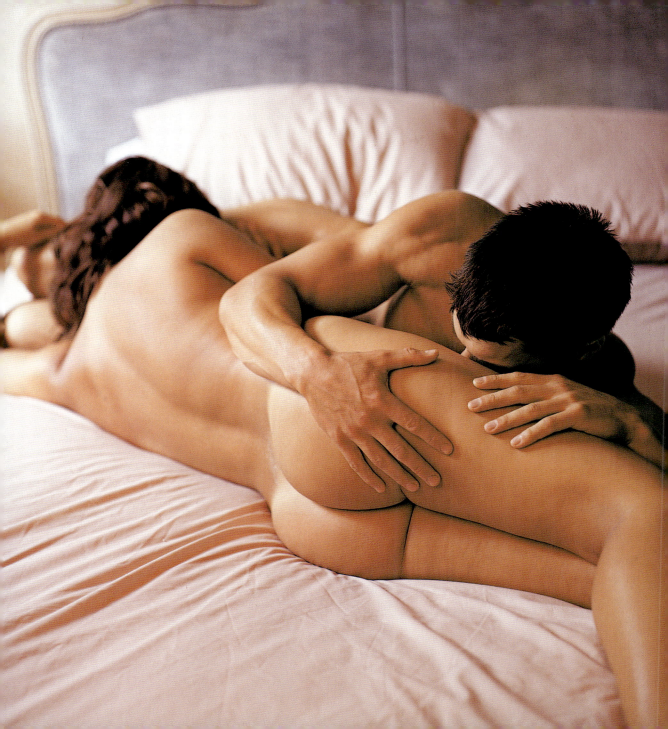

kneel and play

This position feels wonderful because of the contrasting sensations – the slow, intense pressure of your tongue and the light touch of your fingers prepare him for a powerful orgasm. The trick is to take him to the brink and then pull back until his excitement overpowers him. Once you've mastered this technique you can try tying his hands behind his back with a silk scarf so he is completely at your mercy!

all fingers and tongues

With your partner standing, or sitting if this is more comfortable, kneel between his legs. Rub some lube into your hands and tease him a little first. Stroke his tummy, thighs and balls with the lightest of touches – or use a feather for the ultimate in titillation – until he's aroused. To surprise him, and make his toes curl in ecstasy, cool your mouth with some ice, warm it with a hot drink or suck a mint before taking him into your mouth.

candy cane

Flatten your tongue and curve it around his penis just below the tip so that it covers as much of it as possible. Now, slowly wind your tongue around his penis as if licking a stick of candy, keeping your movements slow and firm. Do this three or four times, using the tip of your tongue to tease the glans. Find out where he's most sensitive – it could be on the head or just behind it. Continue to build the pressure: every so often take him out of your mouth and hold him still for a few seconds before fellating him once more until his body ripples with a sensational orgasm.

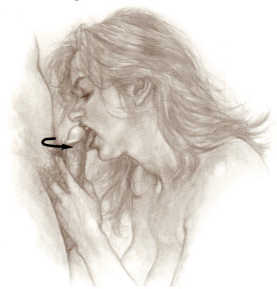

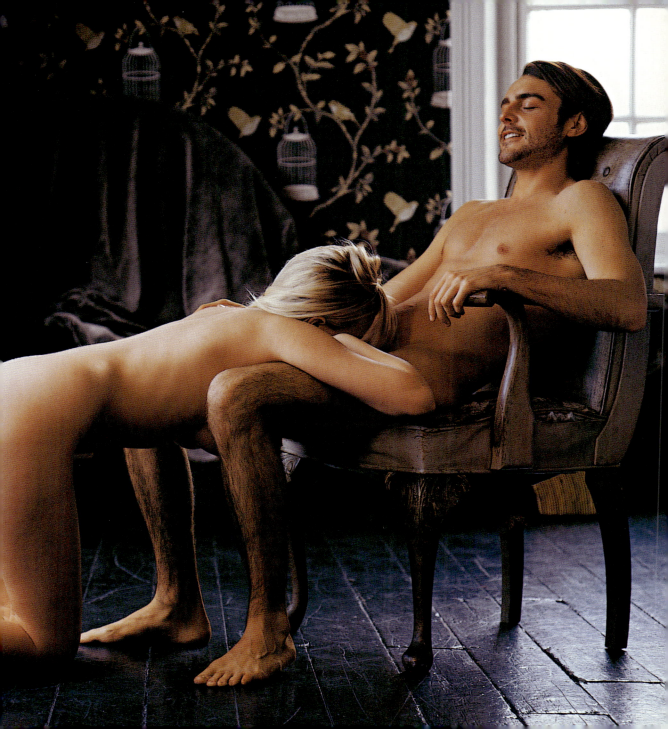

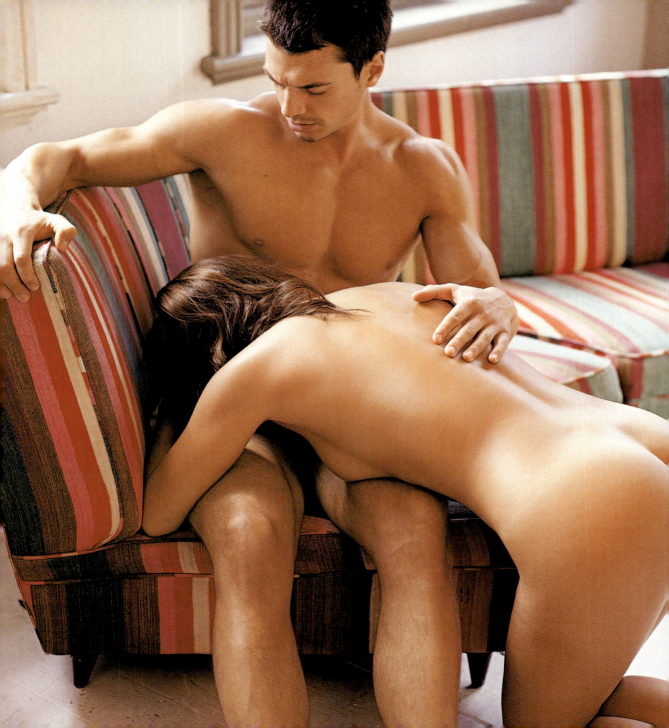

classic with a twist

This position works so beautifully because it's comfortable for you and relaxing for him. It's a classic pose but the twist is that you kneel to one side of him rather than between his legs, allowing you to offer him greater pressure and longer strokes. It also gives you both freedom of movement so that you can tweak his nipples or finger his perineum. And he'll be able to touch you, too, so it's a mutually pleasurable experience. Being able to see what you are doing as well as his expression is a huge turn-on!

ready for action

Get him to sit on the bed or sofa and to lean back slightly while you kneel down with your legs to one side of him. Place a cushion underneath your knees for comfort and rest your arm on his leg for greater stability. Now take his penis in your mouth and hold it there for a moment so he can feel the smooth, wet interior. Once he's hard, start to lick the length of his shaft with both the front and the back of your tongue, so that he can feel the different textures and sensations. Because you're approaching him at an angle, you can move quickly, increasing the pressure until finally he caves into his climax.

> **why not...?**
> *Straddle his legs instead of having them to one side – this pose gives you the chance to stimulate your clitoris at the same time. He'll get twice the pleasure from watching you and being able to fondle your breasts at the same time.*

deepthroat

The idea of deepthroating is that you take his penis beyond your gag reflex so that its entire length is in your mouth. The reason he likes it is because the full length of his penis is being stimulated by your throat as well as your mouth, tongue and lips. He can feel your throat muscles constricting around his penis when you 'gag'. It can be difficult to manage, as most women's jaws are narrower and their throats much shorter than the length of the average penis and it's easier to do if he's got a long penis as opposed to a thick one. However, it's not impossible and with a little practice – and a few tricks – it gets easier.

getting the angle right
Position your partner at the end of the bed while you lie with your head off the edge to take him in backwards. This works perfectly because the angle of his dangle meets the angle of your throat, making it more comfortable to take more of him in. He'll enjoy getting into a rhythm plus there's the psychological aspect of knowing that he's completely inside your mouth.

This position, rather than any other, is good because your throat is at the perfect angle – it has a 90 degree bend and so it's easier to take his penis deeper. For most couples deepthroating takes a lot of practice. Don't feel obliged to keep doing it – if you manage it once in a while that's absolutely fine!

> **why not...?**
> Yawn – not to display boredom but to open your throat muscles. Also, practise the throat and breathing exercises (see pages 60 and 63). If you're turned on, you'll find it much easier to perform so don't use it as a warm up. Keep a glass of water handy as it's easier to do this when your mouth is well lubricated.

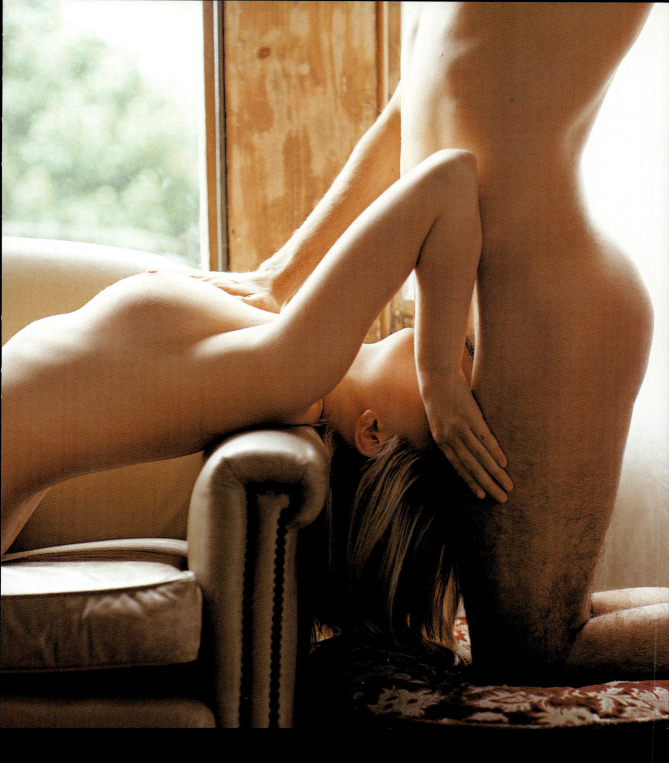

oral–anal play

Also known as analingus or 'rimming', this is very erotic if you're both happy to explore the 'back door'. The anal area is packed with nerve endings and is highly arousing for a man because being touched here stimulates his pelvic floor muscles, which lie beneath the anus. Some people consider it to be 'dirty', so there's the added psychological turn-on of doing something naughty.

on all fours

Ask your partner to get on to all fours on the bed or floor and then kneel down behind him so you can access his buttocks. To practise safe oral sex, use a dental dam or a condom cut in half as a barrier; it helps to add some lube to the inside of the dam – the side facing him – before you start to heighten sensation for him.

Gently lick between his anus from front to back and then change direction. Draw circles with your tongue, using varying levels of pressure. Read his body language and sense what he likes; not all men like it, so ask for feedback. This position is great since you can massage his buttocks and caress his testicles at the same time. If you plan to stimulate him internally, then this is a good way to warm him up and help him relax.

clean him out

If you want to explore anal play but feel a bit squeamish about finding poo, you can clean out his rectal area and reduce the risk of bacterial transmission by giving him a small enema. It's not as scary as it sounds – you gently pump a warm water or herb solution into his anus using a nozzle. Enemas are highly stimulating to some men because they put pressure on the prostate. You can make it a stimulating part of oral sex by doing it creatively.

why not...?

Get him to stand and bend over at the waist while you kneel behind him to reach his buttocks. Alternatively, he could lie on the bed with his knees drawn up; lessen any strain on your neck by raising his body by placing a few cushions underneath him.

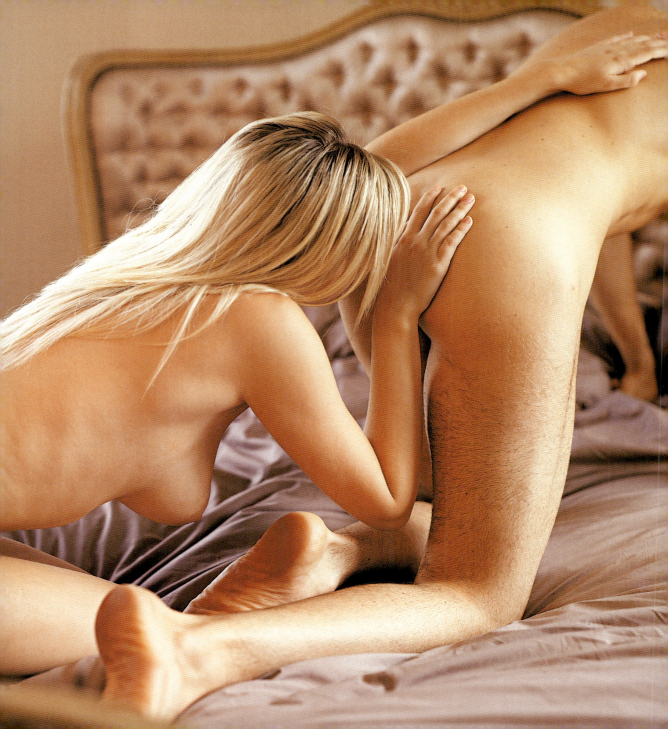

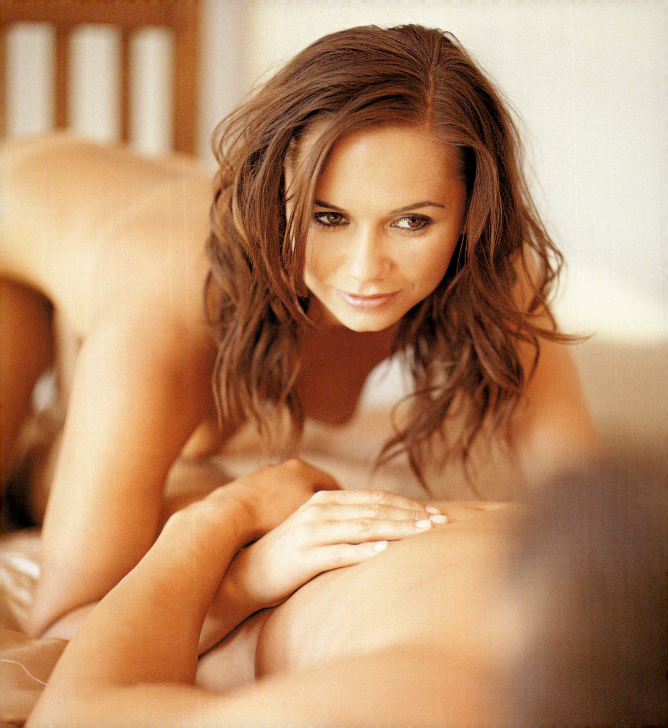

happy endings

To swallow or not to swallow? It's entirely up to you; do what you feel comfortable with. Most men appreciate it if you swallow – it's a sign that you accept them completely. As we explained earlier the consistency and taste of his come can vary but, fortunately, you can use a host of techniques to disguise or change its taste (see page 73).

try this!
Once he's ejaculated don't stop stimulating him straight away. Carry on sucking gently, hum or pulse your hand to his orgasm until he stops and then let go – he'll probably be too sensitive for further stimulation now.

if you love to swallow
You can swallow hard once it's in your mouth and relax your throat so that you hardly taste it. Why not try aiming at different parts of your tongue to change your perception of the taste (see also page 49)? If it's the spurt that puts you off, press on his urethra (at the base of the shaft) as he comes. It won't stop the flow entirely but it may reduce it.

alternative strategies
If you don't want to swallow, quickly take him out of your mouth and finish him off by hand and rub his come into his belly or your cheek, or indeed the rest of your body – always a visual treat for him. If you want to disguise the taste, then try flavoured condoms or lubricant (see also page 114) or numb your tongue with some ice (he'll love that coldness on his cock, too) so that the taste is less noticeable.

have a frank chat
Talk to your partner about how you feel – it's far better than saying nothing and avoiding oral sex simply because you don't like the taste of semen. What is it about it that you dislike? There are ways around most things and there's lots you can do to make it more enjoyable. Relationships are about compromise after all.

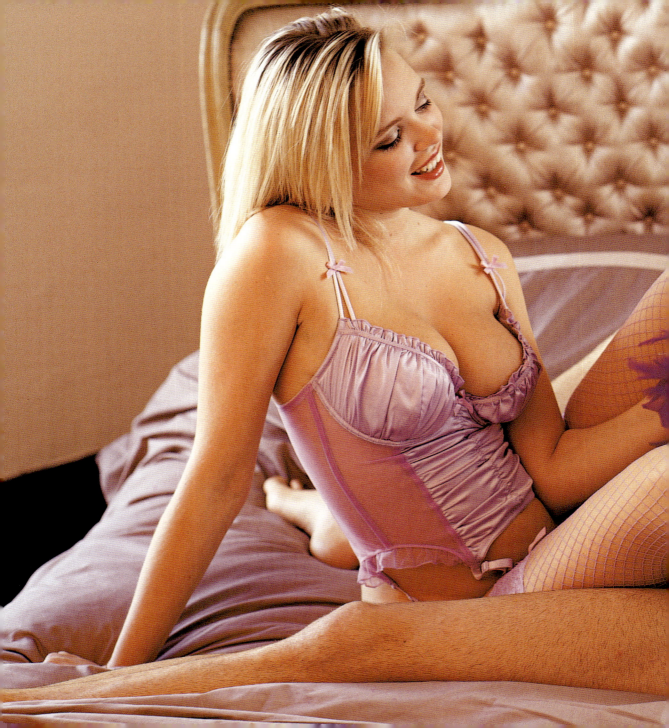

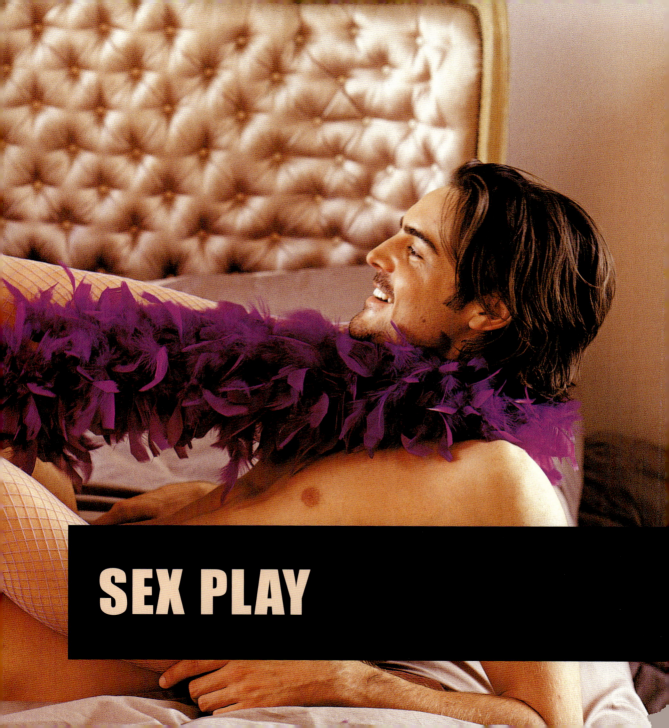

For those of you eager to explore the world of sex play, read on to discover what sex toys are available – and what works best for what – as well as other ideas for spicing up your oral sex life. A tiny change, such as using a prostate massager or switching to a flavoured condom, can reap huge rewards in both the intensity of orgasm and the level of intimacy you share as a couple. So, keep it open and commit to try something new – such as glow-in-the-dark body paint – every once in a while.

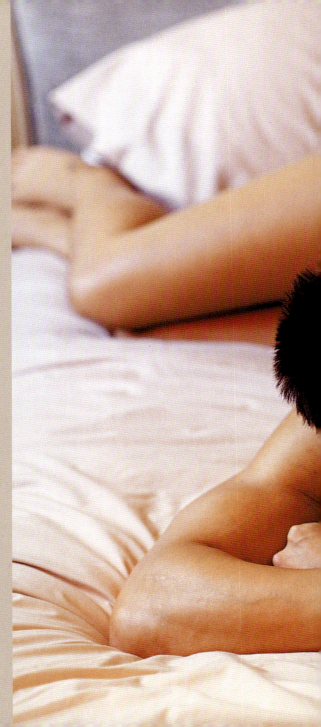

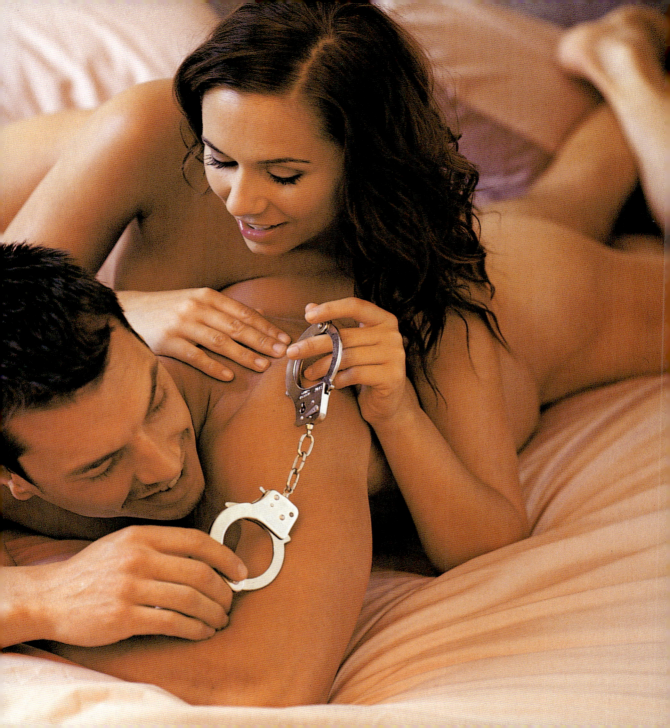

hot accessories

Whether you want to practise safe oral sex or analingus or just want to explore how else you can improve both yours and your partner's experience of fellatio, discover what hot accessories are on the market to help you achieve your goal.

> **try this!**
> Pour some lube on his genitals from way up high for erotic effect, or give him a 'frenchie' – rub some between your breasts and lube him up that way.

all textures, colours and flavours

Condoms come in a wide range of textures – ribbed, super-thin, knobbly or with a special twist – and in an ice-cream van of exciting flavours – strawberry, vanilla, chocolate and tutti frutti to name but a few. Whatever your kink there's probably a condom out there to satisfy it. They are great accessories for fellatio when you don't want to swallow his come.

To find something different shop online or at a sex shop, and get samples to try out various brands. Ultra-thin ribbed ones are a popular choice for oral sex. Lubricated condoms taste foul, instead buy unlubricated ones and add your own lube (make sure it's a water-based one). You can eroticize condoms and make them more fun by using lubricants. Squeezing a drop of lube into the tip before you put it on maximizes his sensation.

dental dams

These thin strips of latex act as a barrier to prevent transmission of bacteria and sexually transmitted infections. You can buy them from a pharmacy or a sex shop, and they are widely used in analingus (always use them for oral–anal play). Not exactly sexy but safe, you can eroticize them by adding lube to intensify the sensation. Try out a few different types of 'wrap' to see what works for you.

smooth and slippery

A must for oral sex. Lubricants make things slippery, sensual and smooth. And there's a host of flavours from good old mint to pina colada. There are several different types: water-based (most widely used as it's compatible with latex and tastes better); oil-based; silicone-based; and 'specialty'.

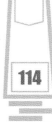

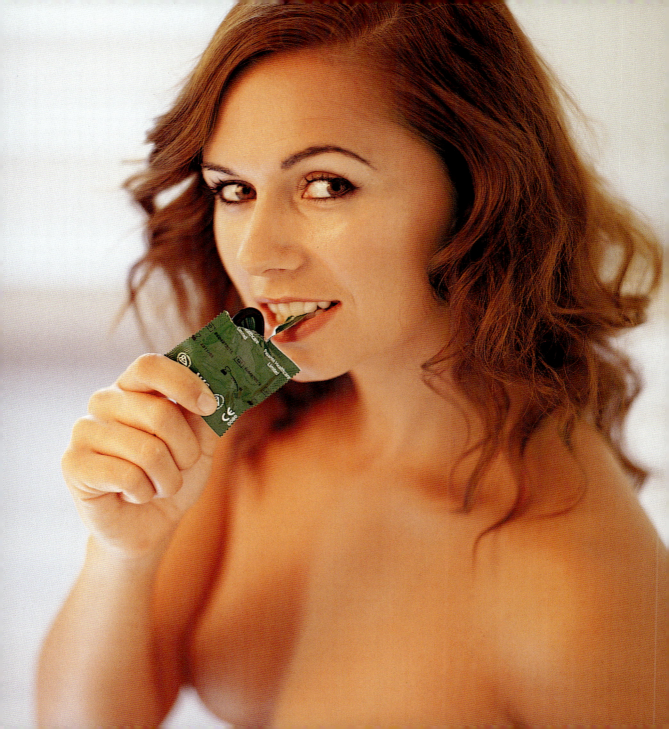

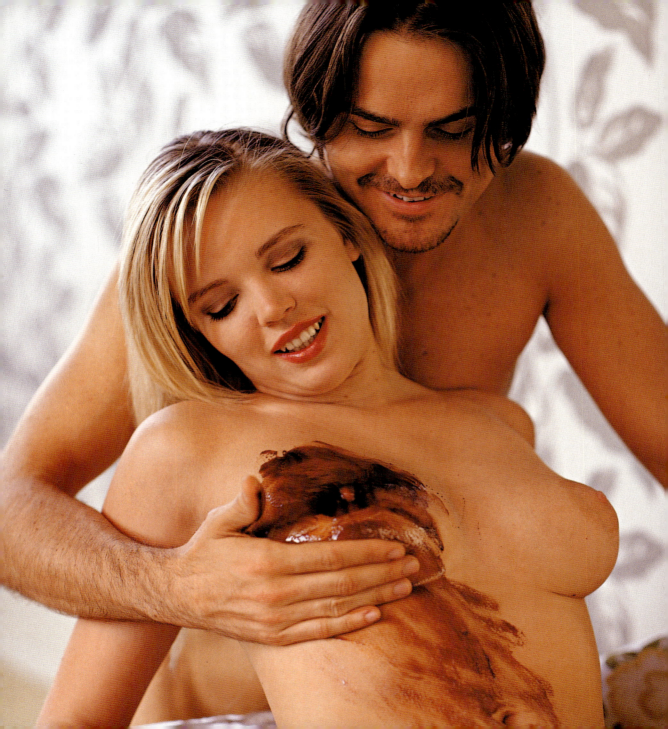

oils, paints and balms

There are lots of fun products to spice up foreplay and oral sex; have a look together online. They add frivolity and spontaneity to sex, and will give you both a few new ideas. Just a couple of rules: if you're using them on his penis then wash off afterwards if you plan to use a condom; and never use them in the vagina as they upset its balance and can lead to yeast infections.

2-in-1 massage oils and lubricants

Some of these oil/lube combinations warm on contact with your body. Plus, they are suitable for external and internal use, which saves the hassle of switching between different types if you want to use them for sex afterwards.

try this!
Cool his penis down by gently massaging some menthol and peppermint oil masturbation balm onto it before your mouth goes on it to warm him up again.

erotic pens and paints

Let out your inner artist. Try drawing or writing messages to one another with these specialist paints and then lick them off. Or, if you fancy a night-time session, why not explore his body under cover with glow-in-the-dark finger paints?

sweeties to suck

If you have a sweet tooth, suck on a candy cock ring (or candy garter or G-string) before oral sex. These sweet somethings will get your juices flowing and make your mouth a hot, wet haven.

nipple gel and cream

Apply some of these to make his (and your) nipples tingle. Sensations can be warm or cooling, depending on what effect you're after.

'love' creams

These creams for genitals contain active ingredients, such as taurine, an amino acid that helps our bodies digest fat, and ginseng, which helps maintain healthy skin and high energy levels, good circulation and a strong erection. Massage a drop on to the tip of his penis to boost his performance and enhance sensation.

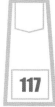

toys for the boys

Toys can be great fun and they can enhance oral sex beyond belief – and they give your hands and mouth a break! The toy market has exploded: there are all manner of toys available – with new ones constantly being developed. Popular toys for use during oral sex include vibrators, dildos, cock-rings and anal toys, such as prostate stimulators and butt plugs.

vibrators

As you'd imagine, vibrators come in all shapes and sizes – dildo-shaped ones, waterproof, prostate or G-spot stimulators, finger vibes and pocket rockets (very popular mini ones that look like a torch). Use them to offer him extra stimulation and improve his orgasms during oral sex. Try using a slim one or a finger vibe against his penis or your mouth while you fellate him for extra vibration. It's wise to check your lubricant is compatible to make it a more sensual experience.

dildos

These penis-shaped toys don't vibrate and are available in a range of materials, such as latex and silicone; like vibrators, you can choose the colour, size and shape of your dildo. Silicone is generally the best quality material to use, as it doesn't smell, holds heat and lasts for ages. Or if you prefer, sample one made of glass – they look and feel fabulous and heat up or cool down according to your preferences so can be fun to use during oral sex sessions or for practice.

butt plugs

You can insert these small toys into your partner's anus or rectum for extra stimulation. Unlike dildos, they have a flared base, which means they can't slip inside him and get lost. Once inside they are held in place by his sphincter muscle. Many men like the sensation of fullness butt plugs provide

> **try this!**
>
> *Position a small vibrator for some extra stimulation between his buttocks during oral sex. Put one on the bed and get him to lie back slowly so that the vibrator nestles between his cheeks.*

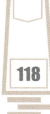

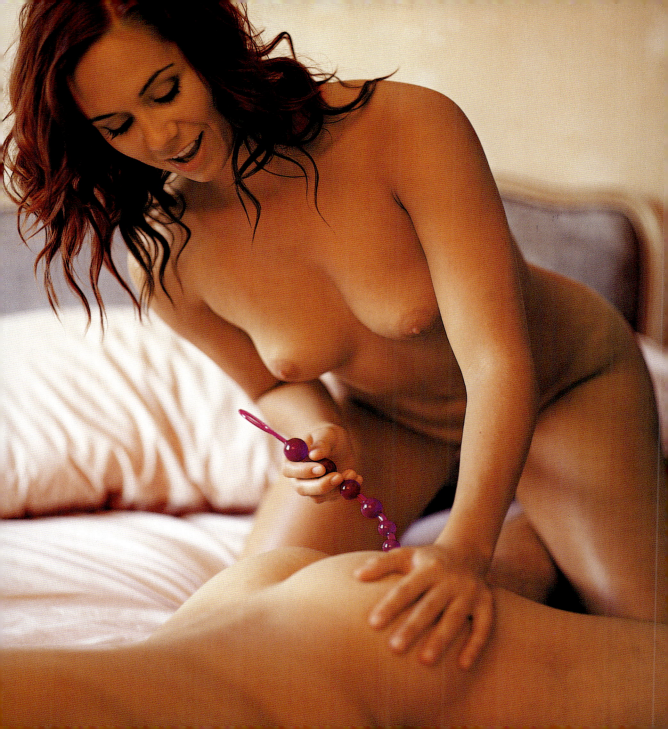

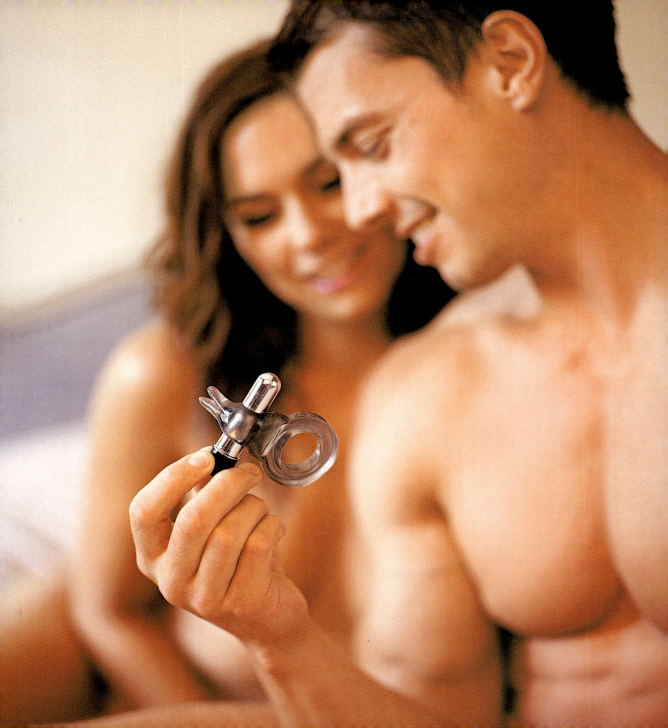

during oral sex. The flared end rubs against his anal area while the tip stimulates his prostate gland, which takes him to a more intense orgasm. If you haven't used one before, choose a small, thin one, use plenty of lube and take your time – he'll thank you for it.

cock-rings

Designed to prolong his erection, cock-rings sit around the base of his penis or scrotum to squeeze the veins and trap blood in the penis – helping him to stay hard for longer. Go for a leather or rope one that you can adjust accordingly. If he likes extra vibration, choose one that has a vibrate option, which will stimulate his balls or his scrotum and perineum. Triple cock-rings have extra attachments to hold the testicles apart so that his orgasm is incredibly intense; but don't use them for extended periods of time.

prostate massagers

These anal toys dip inside the anus to stimulate the prostate gland and can bring your man to orgasm without ejaculation (see page 36). Some are designed to stimulate the anus, prostate and perineum, which gives intense orgasm and can be used to 'milk' his prostate (see page 33). Simpler types look more like a thin dildo with an angled tip. Whichever type you use, lubricate generously and use gentle pressure.

which toy?

When wading through the plethora of sex toys available, how do you know what to choose or try? Firstly, talk about it with your partner and decide what type of sensation you would both like to experience. How convenient does the toy need to be? Do you mind if it's plugged in or do you want to be able to move around? Should it be something that's small, quiet and discreet that you can hold? Then, once you've decided on the toy you'd both like, go shopping for it together.

nipple clamps, pumps and rings

His nipples – like yours – can be quite sensitive so if you haven't already experimented with these give them a try. There are lots of different types on the market so try a few until you find one he likes. They add pressure and vibration to the nipple and restrict blood flow to the area, which makes it more sensitive to touch. A gentle tug during oral sex will feel delicious. Pumps gently 'suck' the nipple delivering a milder sensation while clamps feel more intense if that's what he prefers. They're a fun addition to foreplay that can help to bring him to orgasm more quickly.

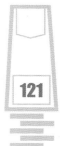

experimenting further

Don't get stuck in a rut, try something new today – whether it's wrapping a silk scarf or a beaded necklace around his penis to give him unusual and fantastic sensations or having a body piercing to intensify your oral technique. Keep him on his toes and experiment.

popular types of genital piercing

Prince Albert – a ring through the bottom of the glans, which heals fairly quickly and looks great.

Hafada – the scrotum is quite painless to pierce; but because of its location, it can easily be caught so it can take longer to heal.

Frenum – this type is popular as it's quick to heal and doesn't hurt much. You pierce the skin underneath the shaft behind the glans.

Foreskin – if he's uncircumcised, he can have one or more piercings here.

Dydoe – in this type, the piercing is at the top or side of the glans; and is mostly for circumcised men.

dressing up

Different fabrics can make foreplay more sensual and exciting. Experiment with leather, latex, PVC, rubber and silk to see which sensations you prefer. Wearing silk knickers while you straddle his leg during oral sex is bound to turn both of you on.

Explore fantasies and play games – whether you desire any man in a uniform or he loves you in that satin strapless number, make the most of your dressing-up time. If you want to play a powerful role, get him to wear a mask or blindfold.

body modification

This ancient practice is a very sensual and erotic way to enhance oral sex. People modify their bodies to promote sexual sensation, as part of BDSM (bondage, discipline, sadism and masochism) or simply to celebrate their diversity and body.

Tongue piercings can heighten the sensations experienced via kissing and licking during oral sex. If you fancy getting your tongue pierced, be warned that it'll take about 4–6 weeks to heal and that you should abstain from oral sexual activities during the healing process. Lip piercings are most commonly seen as a ring or stud through the bottom lip.

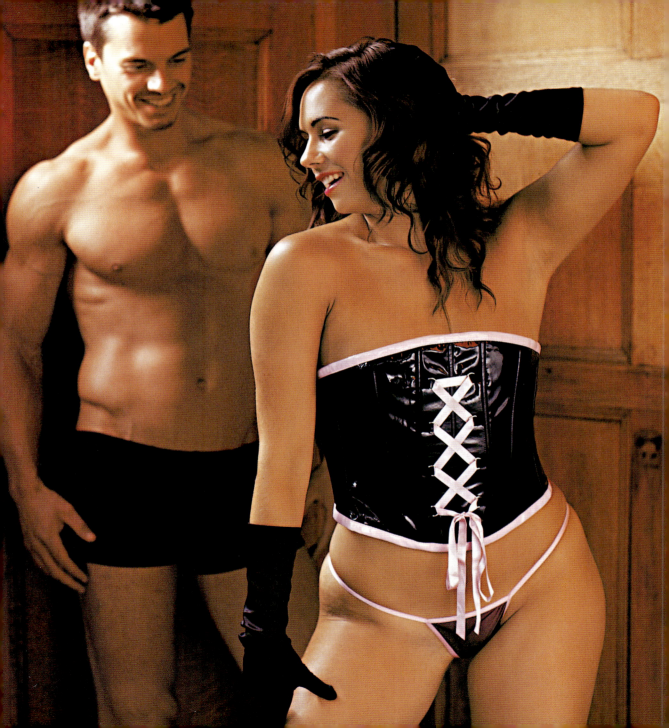

index

A
accessories 114
acupressure 77
alcohol 40, 84
anus 22
    analingus 94, 106, 114
    butt plugs 118–21
    hot spots 30
    prostate massage 33, 121
aphrodisiac foods 73

B
bad breath 50
balls see testicles
bathing together 69
BDSM (bondage, disciple, sadism and masochism) 122
blindfolds 93, 122
blowing 84
body modification 122
body piercing 122
body sushi 73
bondage 122
bones, jaw 49
breasts, 'frenchies' 114
breathing 60
butt plugs 118–21
buttocks
    massage 42
    spanking 88
    using vibrator between 118

C
'candy cane' 100
candy cock rings 117
chairs, erotic 94
chewing gum 59
China 11
chlamydia 14
chocolate 73
circle dance 87
circular breathing 60
circumcision 122
clamps, nipple 121
clitoris 54, 103
clothes 70, 122
cock see penis
cock rings 117, 121
come see ejaculate
condoms
    analingus 106
    flavoured 63, 106, 114
    lubricants and 114
    putting on with tongue 63
    safe sex 14, 106
    textures 114
contraception, withdrawal method 34
coronal ridge 24
corpa cavenosa 34
Cowper's glands 34
creams 117
cuddling 70
cultural differences 11
cunnilingus 93

D
deepthroating 63, 104
dental dams 14, 34, 106, 114
dildos 63, 118
dressing up 122
drugs 40
dydoe piercing 122

E
Egypt, ancient 11
ejaculate
    contents 36
    pre-ejaculate 34, 87
    size of 40
    swallowing 14, 109
    taste of 36, 73, 106
ejaculation see orgasm
ejaculatory ducts 34
endorphins 60, 88
enemas 34, 106
epididymis 34
erection
    problems 27, 29, 40
    stages of 29
erogenous zones 42
erotic furniture 94
erotic massage 77
excitement stage 39
eye contact 70, 90

F
face
    bones 49
    relaxation 57

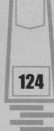

faeces 34, 106
fantasies 70, 94, 122
feathers 100
feet
   massage 42, 77
   reflexology 77
fingers
   as erogenous zone 42
   lacing 88
fish, body sushi 73
flavoured condoms 63, 106, 114
foods, foreplay 73
foot massage 42, 77
foreplay 66–79
foreskin 24, 27
   hygiene 29
   piercings 122
'frenchies' 114
frenulum (sweet spot) 24, 53
   lingam massage 78
   piercings 122
fruit 63, 73
furniture, erotic 94

G
gag reflex 104
games 122
gels 63
genitals
   anatomy 24
   piercing 122
   shaving 69, 74
ginseng 117

glans 24, 27
   piercings 122
   stimulating 87
glass dildos 118
gonorrhoea 14
grinding teeth 57
gum, chewing 59

H
hafada piercing 122
hair, shaving 74
hands
   massaging 42
   techniques 87–90
   tying up 100
   warming 87
head massage 42
heart rate 39
hepatitis 14
herpes 14
HIV 14
hormones 36, 40
hot spots 24, 27, 30, 88
human papilloma virus (HPV) 14
hygiene 29, 34

I J
ice 84, 100, 106
impotence 40
internal massage 33, 121
Isis 11
Japan 97

jaws
   bones 49, 57
   exercise 59
   problems 57

K
kaizen philosophy 97
Kama Sutra 11
Kegel exercises 40
kissing 84
   foreplay 70
   link to clitoris 54
kneeling positions 100–3

L
lacing fingers 88
lesbian porn 70
Lesbos 11
licking 84
linea alba 42
lingam massage 78
lips
   exercises 54
   kissing 54
   muscles 50
   piercings 122
   skin care 54
lipstick 54
'love' creams 117
lubricants
   and condoms 114
   flavoured 63, 106, 114
   'frenchies' 114

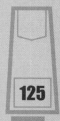

2-in-1 massage oils and lubricants 117

M
mandible bone 49, 57
masks 122
masochism 122
massage
    erotic massage 77
    lingam massage 78
    oils 117
    prostate massage 33, 121
Masters and Johnson 39
masturbation 27
masturbation balm 117
maxillae bones 49
meatus 24
meditation 60
menthol 117
meridians, acupressure 77
'milking' prostate gland 33, 121
million-dollar point 22, 30, 84
mirrors 93
mobile phones 70
mouth
    exercises 50
    lips 54
multiple orgasms 36
muscles
    jaw exercises 59
    orgasm 36
    pelvic floor exercises 40
    pubococcygeus (PC) muscle 33
    tongue 49
music 70
myths 12

N
nail care 70
nakedness 69

neck exercises 59
nibbling 54
nipples
    excitement 39
    nipple gel 117
    sex toys 121
    stimulating 42

O
oils, massage 117
orgasm 36, 39–40
    delaying 90
    multiple orgasms 36
    'organ' orgasms 78
    premature ejaculation 40
    prostate orgasm 33
    without ejaculation 36
Osiris 11

P
paints 117
papillae 49
pelvic floor exercises 40
penis 20–7
    anatomy 24
    cock rings 117, 121
    corpa cavenosa 34
    erection problems 27, 29, 40
    face-sitting 94
    hand techniques 87
    handling 27
    kissing 84
    lingam massage 78
    piercings 122
    size 24
    stages of erection 29
    underside of 88
pens, erotic 117
peppermint oil 117
perineum 22, 30, 84
phenylethylamine 73

phones 70
piercings 122
pituitary gland 40
plateau stage 39
porn 70
positions 82
    classic with a twist 103
    deepthroating 104
    kneeling positions 100
    oral-anal play 106
    shoulder stand 97
    sixty-nine 98
    the warrior 93
practice 63
pre-ejaculate 34, 87
premature ejaculation 40
prick tease 90
Prince Albert piercing 122
problems 12, 27, 29, 40
prolactin 40
prostate gland 33, 34
    butt plugs 121
    enemas and 106
    massagers 121
    orgasm 33
    stimulating 30, 33, 84, 90
prostitutes 14
pubic bone 22
pubic hair, shaving 74
pubococcygeus (PC) muscle 33
pump technique 88
pumps, nipple 121

Q
quickies 90
    frenulum 24
    saliva 53
    sixty-nine 98
    standing positions 93

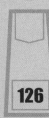

R
razors 74
reflexology 77, 78
refractory period 40
relaxation 57, 60, 77
resolution stage 40
rhythm 27, 84
rimming 94, 106

S
sadism 122
safe sex 14
saliva 53, 84
scalp massage 42
scrotum 22, 30
   cock rings 121
   piercings 122
   shaving 74
semen 33, 34, 36
   taste of 36, 73, 106
seminal fluid 34
seminal vesicles 34
serotonin 73
sex play 111–23
sexual response, stages of 39–40
sexually transmitted infections (STIs) 14
shaft, handling 27
shaving genitals 69, 74
shoulder stand 97
silicone dildos 63, 118
singing 60
sitting, on face 94
sixty-nine position 98
skin
   as erogenous zone 42
   semen and 36
sleep 36, 40
smegma 29
smells 29
smoking 49
soixante-neuf position 98
spanking 88
speaking, jaw exercises 59
sperm 34, 36
squeeze and hold technique 87
standing positions 93, 98
stimulation, stages of 39
stomach massage 42
stress 57
sushi 73
swallowing ejaculate 14, 109
sweet spot *see* frenulum
syphilis 14

T
Taoism 29, 30, 70, 78
taste buds 49
taste of semen 36, 73, 106
taurine 117
'tea bagging' 84
teasing 27, 90
teeth
   grinding 57
   nibbling 54
   unzipping trousers with 93
temporal bone 49
testicles 22, 30
   cock rings 121
   'tea bagging' 84
testosterone 39–40
thigh massage 42
throat, deepthroating 63, 104
toes, as erogenous zone 42
tongue
   brushing 50
   'candy cane' 100
   exercises 50
   muscles 49
   papillae 49
   piercings 122
   putting condoms on with 63
   sensitivity 49
toys 69, 118–21
trousers, unzipping with teeth 93
tryptophan 73

U V
urethra 24
urine 24
vas deferens 34
vegetables, practising with 63
vibrators 118, 121

W Y
'wand of light' 78
the warrior 93
withdrawal method, contraception 34
worries 12, 29
yin and yang 77

acknowledgements

Author acknowledgements
Thanks to: Laura MacDonald at NORM-UK; Alexandra Obrado! vich, reflexologist; Charlie Gluckman, staff sexologist at Good Vibrations; Dr Patrick French, GUM Consultant; Monique Carty at sextoys.co.uk; Sonia Marshall at Myriad PR; milkymoments foreplay; Suzanne Noble, Noble PR; Sarah Hedley, Suzanne Portnoy, and everyone else who shared their oral tips and tricks.

Publisher acknowledgements
Executive Editor: Jane McIntosh
Managing Editor: Clare Churly
Deputy Creative Director: Karen Sawyer
Designer: Peter Gerrish
Photographer: John Davis
Illustrator: Patricia Ludlow @ Linden Artists
Production Controller: Nigel Reid